NO NEED FOR *seconds*

Nicholas Kelly, MS, RD, LD

Photos By Jiajia Huang

TABLE OF CONTENTS

BREAKFAST RECIPES

LUNCH

DINNER

DINNER SIDES

SNACKS

SOUPS

DESSERTS

BEVERAGES

Nutritional facts for each recipe are at the end of each section.

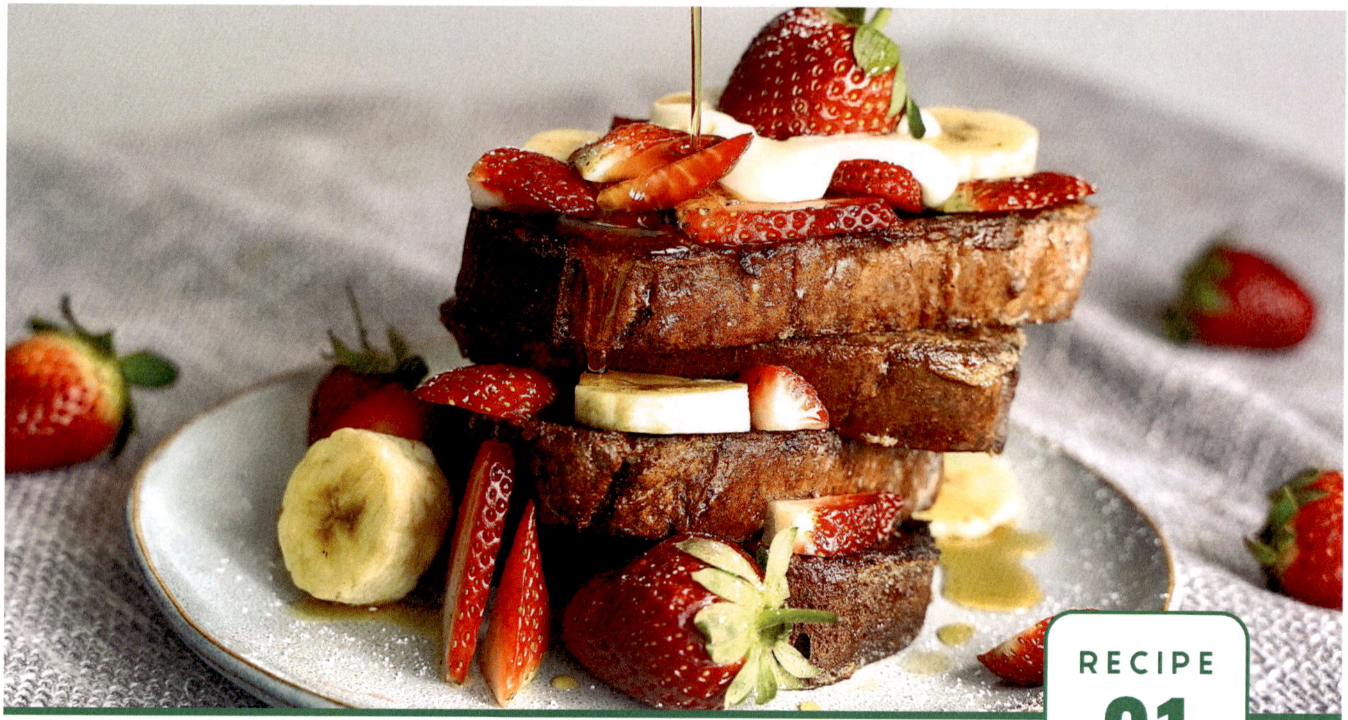

BANANA BREAD FRENCH TOAST

RECIPE 01

INGREDIENTS

BANANA BREAD

2 cups all-purpose flour (250g)
3/4 cup granulated sugar (150g)
3/4 teaspoon baking soda (3.5g)
1/2 teaspoon salt (3g)
1½ cups peeled and mashed ripe bananas - (337.5g)
1/4 cup whole milk (61g)
2 jumbo eggs (126g)

INGREDIENTS

FRENCH TOAST

3 jumbo eggs (189g)
3/4 cup whole milk (183g) - or 1/2 cup heavy cream (118.3g)
1 teaspoon vanilla extract (4.2g)
2 teaspoons cinnamon (5.2g)
2 tablespoons unsalted butter (28.4g)
2 tablespoons canola oil (28g)

INGREDIENTS

GARNISH

1/4 cup maple syrup (56.7g)- or 1/4 cup pancake syrup, such as Mrs. Butterworth's (78.5g)
1 cup sliced strawberries (166g)
1 tablespoon fresh whipped cream (3g)

PREPARATION

BANANA BREAD:

1. Preheat oven to 350°F (175°C). Lightly grease a non-stick 9x5-inch loaf pan.
2. Add the flour, sugar, baking soda and salt to a large bowl and mix.
3. In another large bowl, add the mashed bananas, whole milk and eggs, whisk until smooth.
4. Carefully fold the flour mixture into the banana mixture until well combined. Be careful not to over-mix.
5. Scrape the batter into a non-stick 9x5-inch loaf pan. Bake for 55 minutes, or until a toothpick comes out clean when inserted in the center of the loaf.
6. Allow the banana bread to completely cool, and then cut into 1-inch-thick slices.

FRENCH TOAST:

1. In a medium bowl, whisk the eggs, whole milk or cream, vanilla, and cinnamon.
2. In a large, shallow skillet over medium heat, add butter and canola oil and heat until the butter is melted.
3. Once the butter and oil are heated, dip four slices of banana bread into the egg-milk mixture, coating each side. Allow any excess mixture to drip off.
4. Place the slices in the skillet and cook for 3 minutes on each side or until browned.
5. Transfer the finished French toast slices to a plate, and repeat until you've made the amount of French toast you desire.
6. Serve with the garnishes and enjoy.

*Note: *The longer you let the banana bread soak in the liquid mixture, the more moist it will become. You can even let it soak overnight to obtain an extra moist product.**

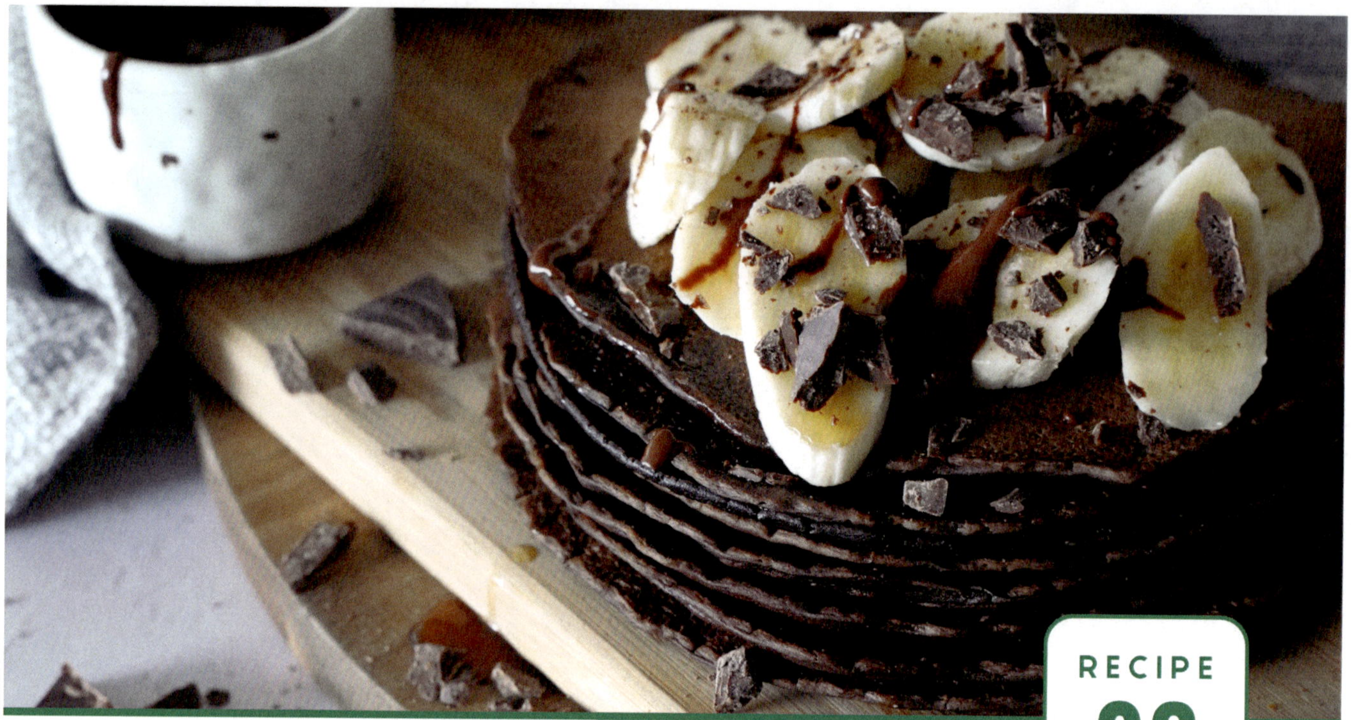

RECIPE 02

HOT CHOCOLATE PANCAKES

INGREDIENTS

1 cup all-purpose flour (125g)
4 tablespoons unsweetened cocoa powder (21.6g)
2 tablespoons granulated sugar (25.2g)
1 teaspoon baking soda (4.6g)
1/4 teaspoon kosher salt (1.5g)
1/2 teaspoon vanilla extract (2.1g)
1 jumbo egg (63g)
1 cup whole milk (244g)
1/4 cup water (59.3g)
2 tablespoons canola oil (28g)

*Note: *For fluffier pancakes add an additional 1/2 teaspoon of baking soda**

INGREDIENTS

GARNISH

1 cup ripe banana slices (150g)
1/4 cup pancake syrup, such as Mrs. Butterworth's (78.5g)
2 tablespoons caramel syrup (40g)
2 tablespoons chocolate syrup (39g)
1/3 cup miniature marshmallows (15g)
1/2 oz. marshmallow cream (14.2g)
1 tablespoon fresh whipped cream (3g)

PREPARATION

1. In a large bowl, whisk the flour, cocoa powder, sugar, baking soda and salt together.
2. In another bowl, whisk the vanilla, egg, whole milk, water, and canola oil together until well combined.
3. Add the dry mixture to the wet mixture and mix gently until a few lumps remain. Avoid over-mixing, as it will create tough pancakes.
4. Allow the batter to rest for at least 5 minutes. The longer the batter rests (up to 30 minutes), the fluffier the pancakes will be.
5. Place a non-stick skillet over medium-low heat. When hot, pour the batter into the pan in 1/4 cup portions.
6. Cook the pancakes until they have bubbles throughout their entire surface.
7. Flip the pancakes and cook for an additional minute and a half, or until golden brown, and a toothpick inserted in the center of a pancake comes out clean.
8. Transfer the pancakes to a large plate. Add garnishes as desired, serve, and enjoy.

*Note: *If the skillet is not non-stick, coat the pan with butter, oil, or non-stick spray**

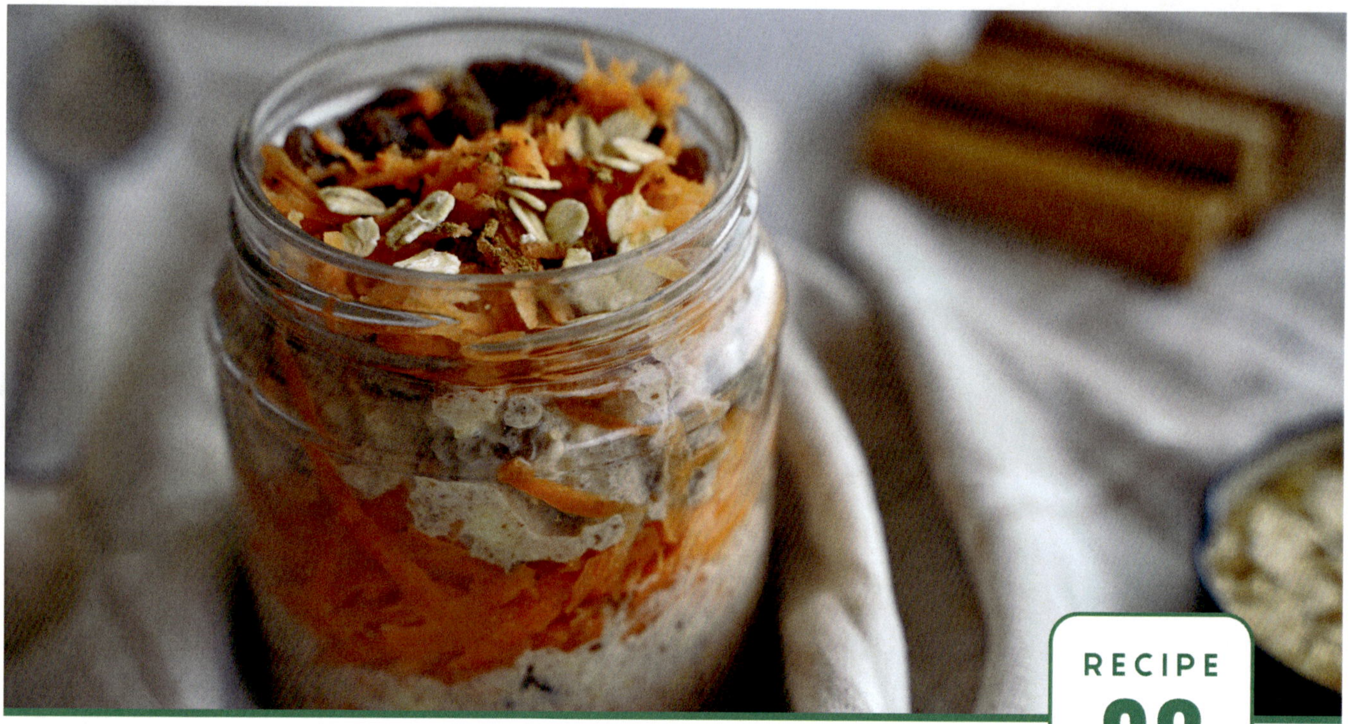

RECIPE 03

CARROT CAKE

INGREDIENTS

- 1/3 cup rolled oats (26.7g)
- 1 tablespoon flax meal (6.5g)
- 1/2 teaspoon cinnamon (1.3g)
- 1/2 cup shredded carrots (61g)
- 1/4 cup raisins (41.3g)
- 1/2 cup whole milk - (122g) for a thick consistency, or 2/3 cup (163g) for a thinner consistency
- 1/3 cup Greek yogurt (56.1g)
- 1/2 teaspoon vanilla extract (2.1g)

PREPARATION

1. In a jar or small bowl with a lid, combine the oats, flax meal, cinnamon, carrots, and raisins and mix.
2. Add the milk, Greek yogurt, vanilla and mix well.
3. Once the ingredients are thoroughly mixed, press the oats down with a spoon to ensure they are moistened and immersed in liquid.
4. Cover securely with a lid and place in the refrigerator overnight, or for at least 6 hours, to set/soak.
5. Remove from the refrigerator, stir, and enjoy.

*Note: *Oats can be microwaved for 30 seconds to 1 minute if warm oats are preferred**

NOTES:

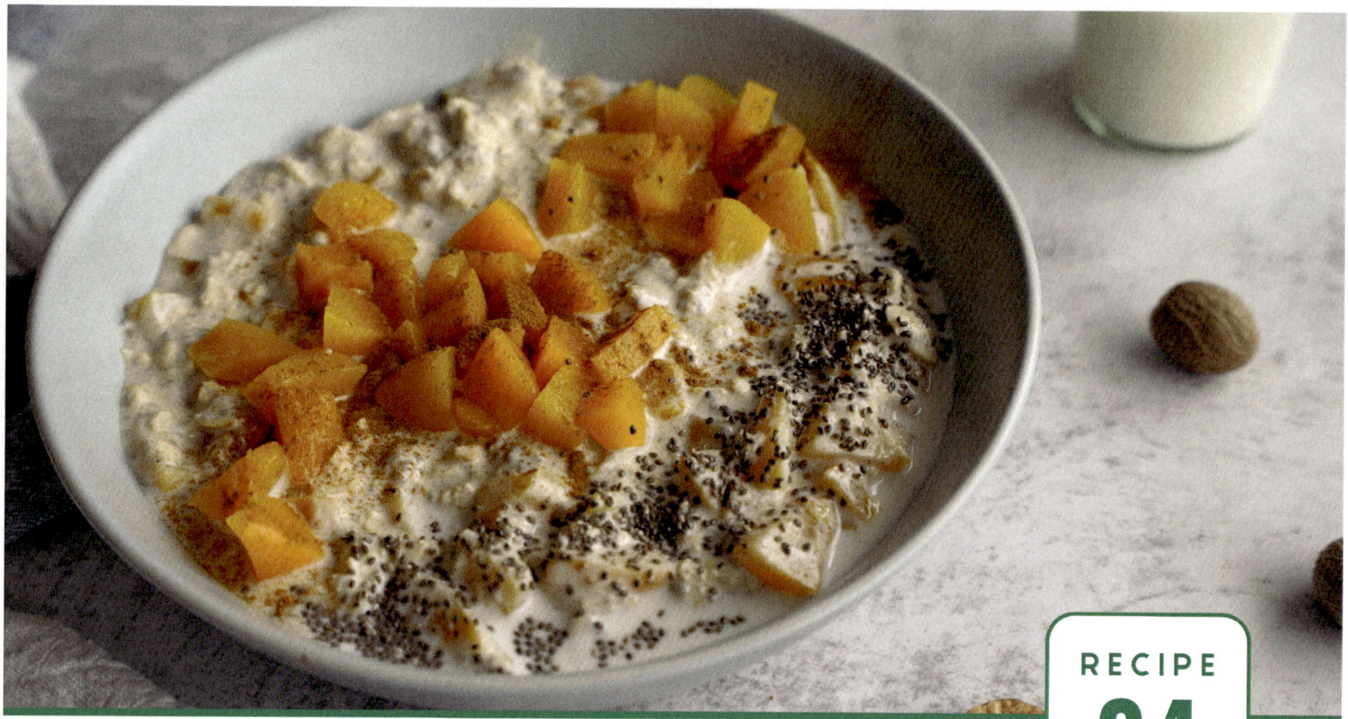

RECIPE 04

PEACHY CLEAN

INGREDIENTS

1/3 cup rolled oats (26.7g)
1/2 teaspoon cinnamon (1.3g)
1/2 teaspoon nutmeg (3.5g)
Pinch of salt
1 tablespoon chia seeds (12g)

1/2 cup whole milk - (122g) for a thick consistency, or 2/3 cup (163g) for a thinner consistency
1/3 cup Greek yogurt (56.1g)
2 tablespoons maple syrup (28.4g)
1/2 teaspoon vanilla extract (2.1g)
1/2 cup chopped peaches (225g)

PREPARATION

1. In a jar or small bowl with a lid, combine the oats, cinnamon, nutmeg, salt, chia seeds and mix.
2. Add the milk, Greek yogurt, maple syrup, vanilla extract, peaches and mix well.
3. Once the ingredients are thoroughly mixed, press the oats down with a spoon to ensure they are moistened and immersed in liquid.
4. Cover securely with a lid and place in the refrigerator overnight, or for at least 6 hours, to set/soak.
5. Remove from the refrigerator, stir, and enjoy.

*Note: *Oats can be microwaved for 30 seconds to 1 minute if warm oats are preferred**

NOTES:

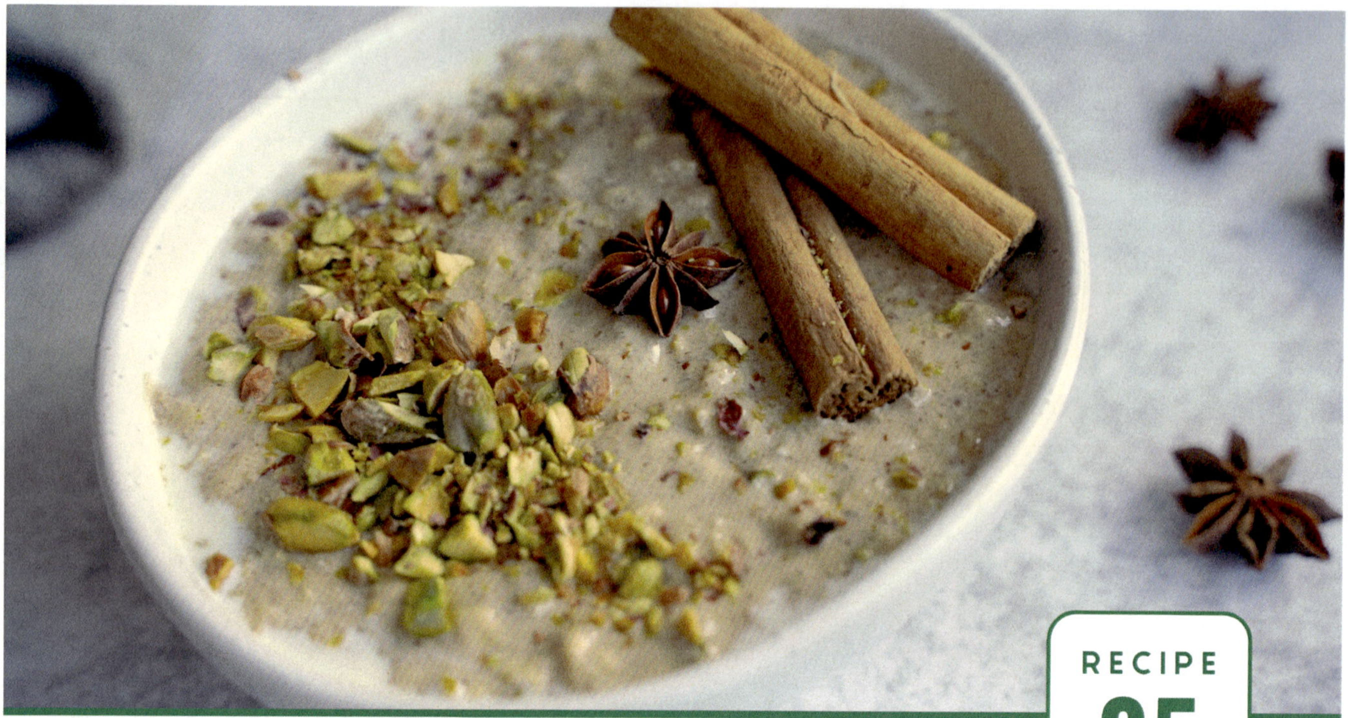

RECIPE 05

CHAI'D AND TRUE

INGREDIENTS

1/3 cup rolled oats (26.7g)
1 tablespoon flax meal (6.5g)
16 shelled pistachios (11.2g)
2 tablespoons chai spice mix (18g)

1/2 cup whole milk – (122g) for a thick consistency, or 2/3 cups (163g) for a thinner consistency
1/3 cup Greek yogurt (56.1g)
2 teaspoons vanilla extract (8.4g)
2 tablespoons maple syrup (28.4g)

PREPARATION

1. In a jar or small bowl with a lid, combine the oats, flax meal, pistachios, and chai spice and mix.
2. Add the milk, Greek yogurt, vanilla extract and maple syrup and mix well.
3. Once the ingredients are thoroughly mixed, press the oats down with a spoon to ensure they are moistened and immersed in liquid.
4. Cover securely with a lid and place in the refrigerator overnight, or for at least 6 hours, to set/soak.
5. Remove from the refrigerator, stir, and enjoy.

*Note: *Oats can be microwaved for 30 seconds to 1 minute if warm oats are preferred**

NOTES:

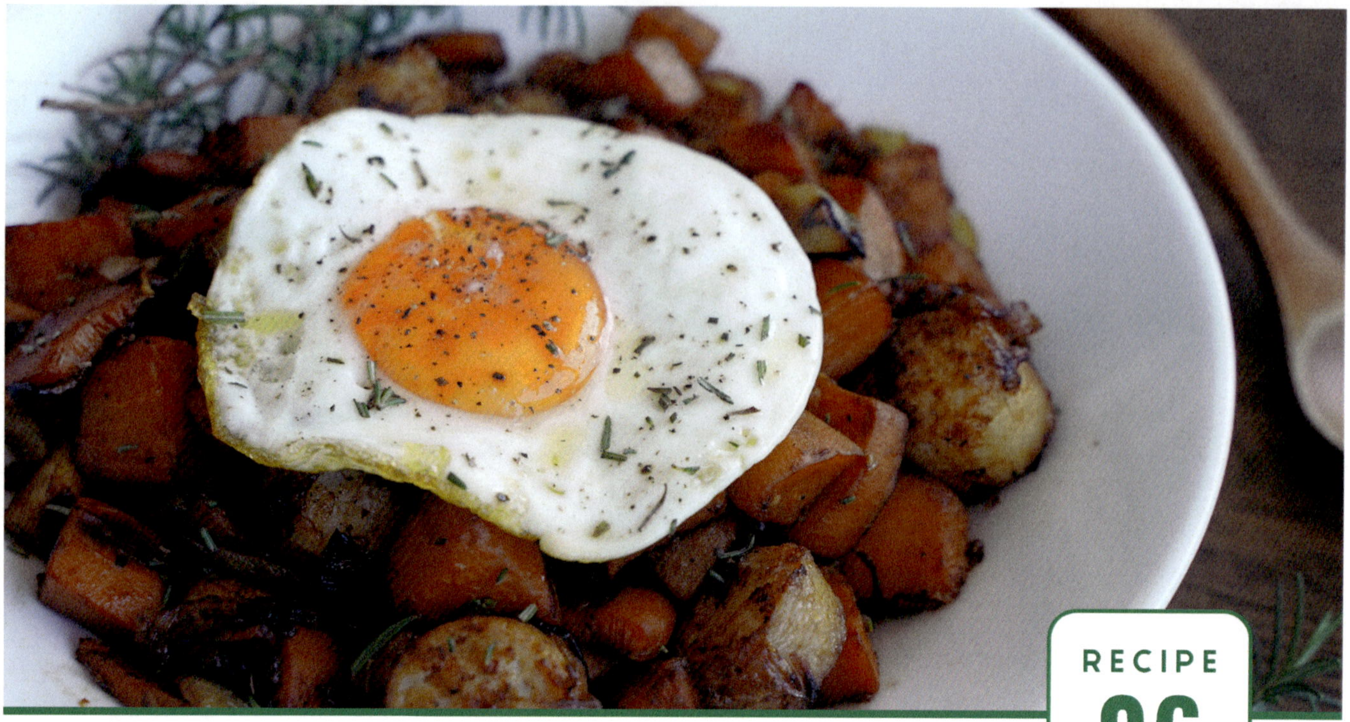

RECIPE 06

SWEET POTATO HASH WITH SUNNY-SIDE UP EGG

INGREDIENTS

SWEET POTATO

1 tablespoon unsalted butter (14.2g)
or canola oil (4.6g)
1 cup diced yellow onion (87g)
2 oz. smoked turkey Italian sausage (56.7g)
3 cups peeled and diced sweet potatoes (399g)
1 tablespoon garlic powder (9.7g)
1 teaspoon kosher salt (6.0g)
1 teaspoon black pepper (2.3g)
1 teaspoon chopped fresh rosemary (1.7g)

INGREDIENTS

SUNNY-SIDE UP EGG

1/2 tablespoon unsalted butter (7.1g)
1 teaspoon extra-virgin olive oil (4.6g)
1 jumbo egg (63g)
1/2 teaspoon salt (3g)
1/2 teaspoon black pepper (1.2g)

PREPARATION

POTATO HASH:

1. In a large skillet over medium heat, melt butter or heat oil. Add the onions and cook, stirring occasionally, until the onions soften.
2. Add the Italian sausage and cook, stirring and breaking it apart until it browns.
3. When cooked, transfer the onions and sausage to a plate and set aside. The oil left after cooking the onions and sausage should be left in the pan while removing the onions and sausage.
4. Place sweet potatoes in the pan used for the onions and sausage. Turn the heat to medium-low, cover with a lid and cook for 10 minutes.
5. Remove the lid, sprinkle the garlic powder, kosher salt, black pepper and rosemary over the potatoes, and stir to coat. Cook for 5 minutes, flipping the potatoes over as they brown. Repeat 3 times.
6. Return the onions and sausage to the pan and increase the heat to medium. Cook for an additional 5 minutes to heat the onions and sausage and allow flavors to blend with the potatoes. Once heated through, remove from the heat and cover until ready to serve.

EGG:

1. Place the butter and olive oil in a medium skillet over low heat until the butter is melted.
2. Crack the egg into a bowl, and then gently pour the egg into the skillet.
3. Cover the skillet with a lid and cook, undisturbed, until the white is completely set, but the yolk is still runny, about 2 to 2½ minutes.
4. Season with salt and pepper. Transfer the egg to a plate and add a scoop of the sweet potato hash. Serve and enjoy.

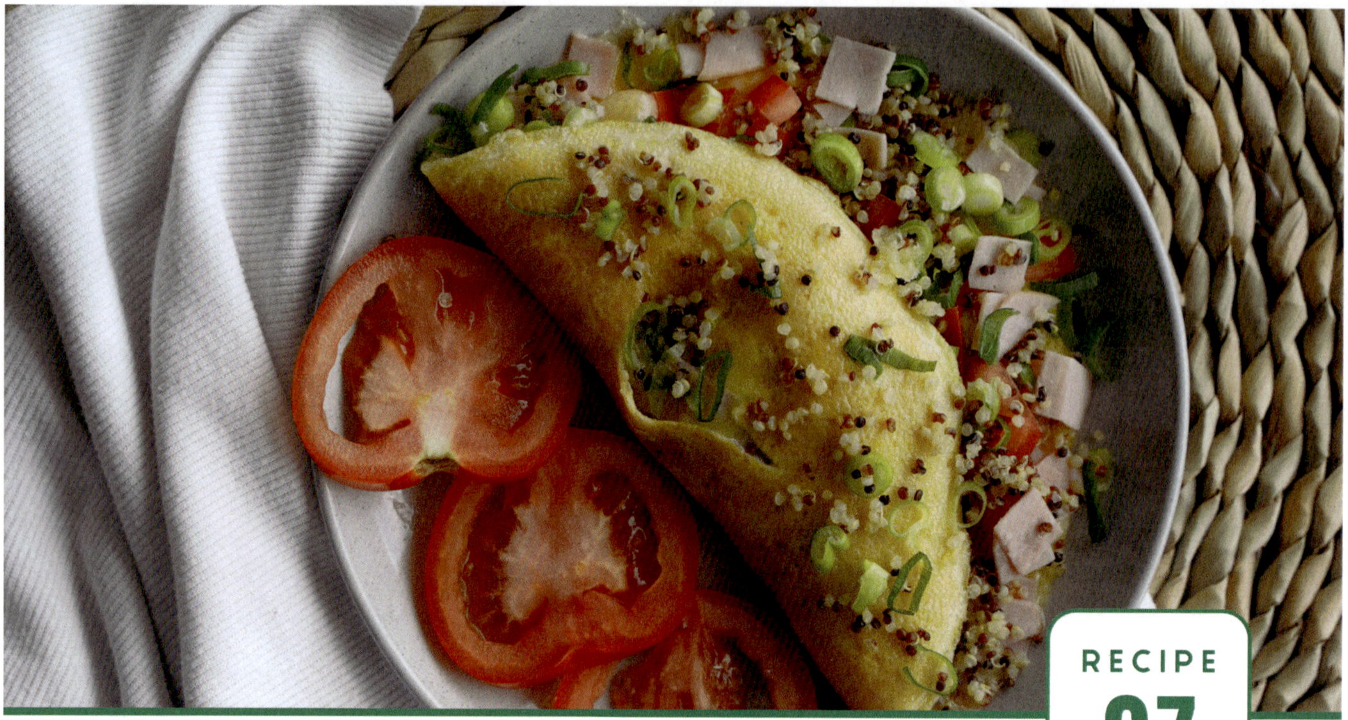

RECIPE 07

EASY OMELET WITH FLAIR

INGREDIENTS

BULK UP

1/2 cup cooked quinoa (92.5g)
1/4 cup chopped ham (56.7g)
1/4 cup green onion (17.8g)
1/4 cup chopped tomato (45g)
3/4 cup shredded cheddar cheese (56.5g)
1 tablespoon Cajun seasoning (14.2g)

INGREDIENTS

SOUTHWEST

1/4 cup salsa (64.8g)
3/4 cup chopped avocado (112.5g)
1/4 cup chopped white mushroom (40g)
1/4 cup chopped red bell pepper (37.3g)
1/4 cup chopped white onion (40g)
1 tablespoon chopped cilantro (14.2g)
1/2 cup shredded Swiss cheese (54g)
A squeeze of fresh lime juice

INGREDIENTS

VEGGIE

1/4 cup chopped roasted eggplant (20.5g)
1/4 cup chopped roasted squash (51.2g)
1/4 cup chopped red onion (37g)
1/4 cup broccoli florets (22.8g)
1/4 cup chopped tomato (45g)
3/4 cup shredded provolone cheese (99g)

TOPPING COMBINATIONS

Vegetables can be cooked or raw for omelets; however, meat must be cooked before adding it to omelets.

INGREDIENTS

2 jumbo eggs (126g)
1/2 tablespoon unsalted butter (7.1g)
Pinch of salt

PREPARATION

1. Whisk the eggs and salt until the egg yolk and egg white are completely mixed.
2. In a medium skillet over medium-high heat, melt the butter. Pour the egg mixture into the pan. It should begin to bubble immediately.
3. After 30 seconds, carefully flip the omelet over using a wide spatula. Top with your desired vegetables and protein, making sure they are evenly distributed.
4. Cook for another 30 seconds and fold over. Serve and enjoy.

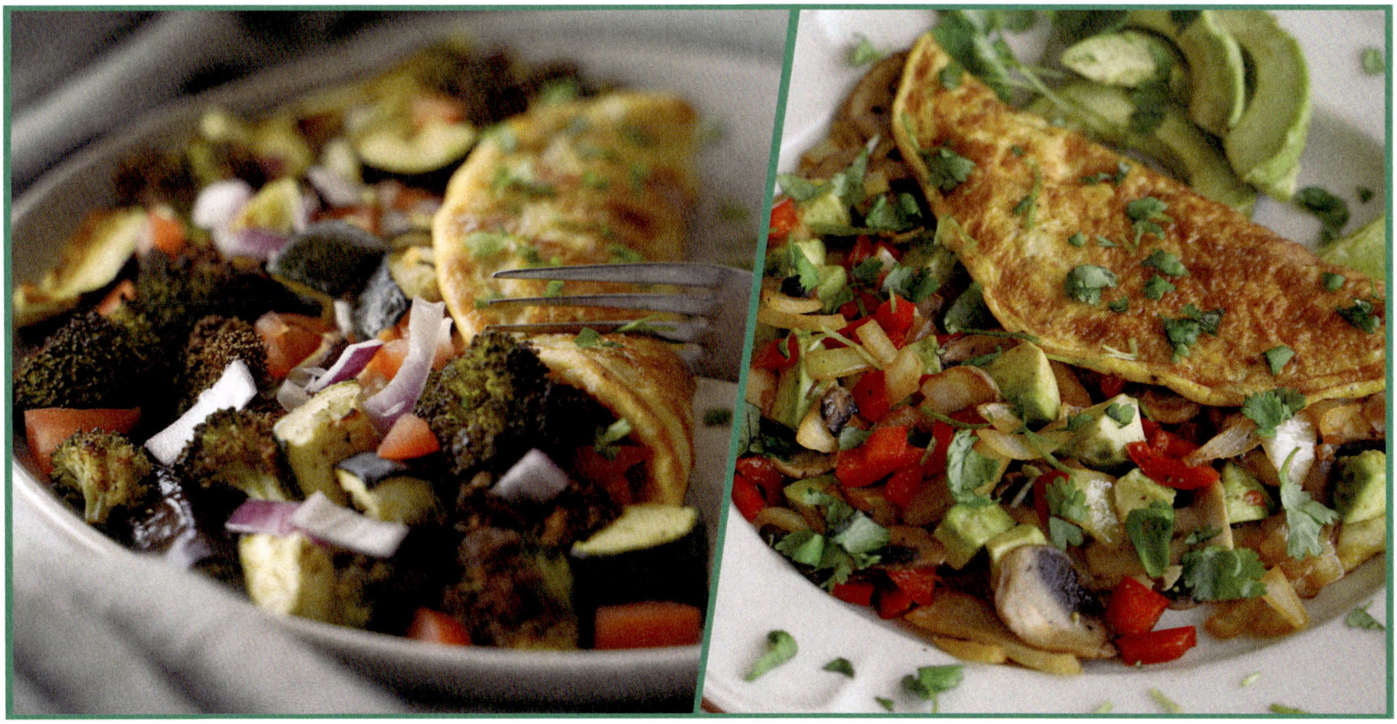

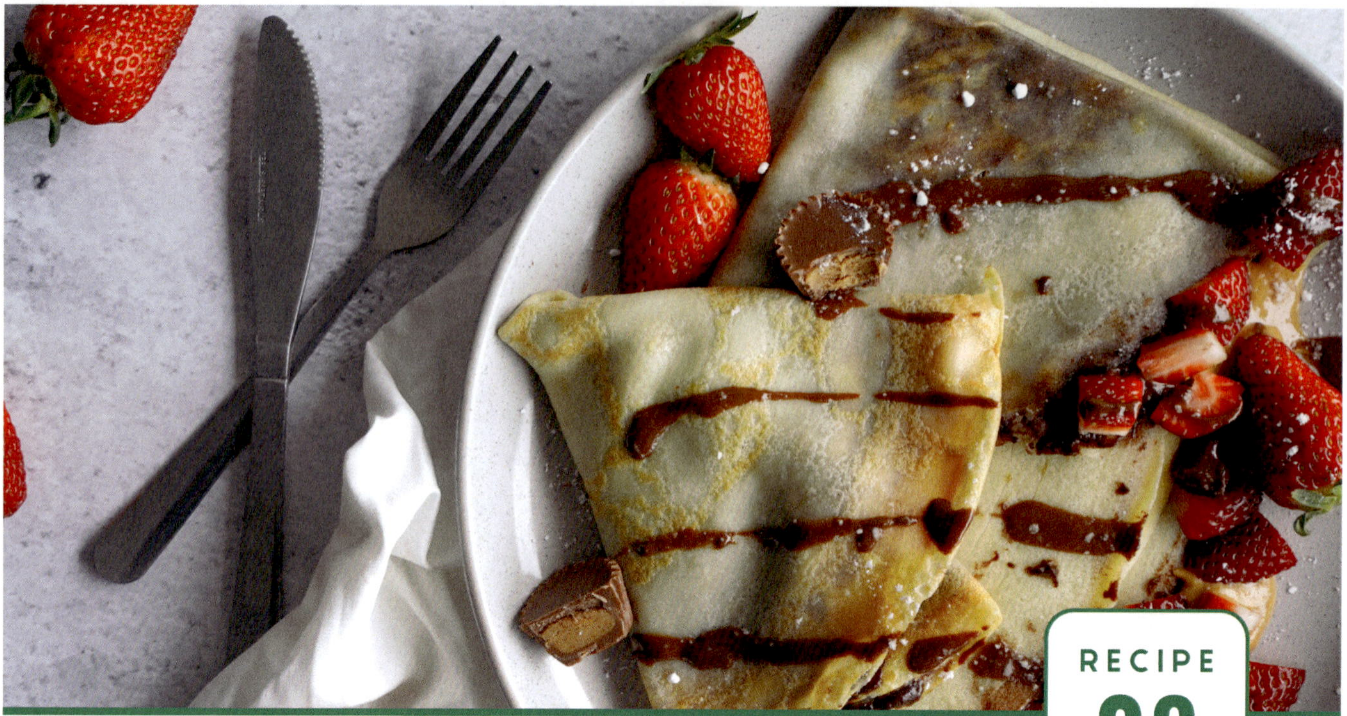

RECIPE
08

REESE'S PEANUT BUTTER CREPES

INGREDIENTS

1 cup all-purpose flour (125g)
2 jumbo eggs (126g)
1/2 cup whole milk (122g)
1/2 cup water (118.5g)
1/4 teaspoon salt (1.5g)
2 tablespoons unsalted butter - melted (28.4g)
1/2 tablespoon Nutella hazelnut chocolate spread (18.5g)
1/2 tablespoon smooth peanut butter (16g)

PREPARATION

1. Heat a lightly oiled griddle or frying pan over medium-high heat. In a large bowl, whisk the flour and eggs together.
2. Gradually add the whole milk, then the water, stirring continually to combine.
3. Add the salt and butter and beat until smooth.
4. Pour or scoop the batter onto the griddle or frying pan, using approximately 1/4 cup for each crepe.
5. Tilt the pan in a circular motion so that the batter coats the surface evenly. Cook the crepe for about 2 minutes or until the bottom is light brown. Loosen gently with a spatula, flip, and cook the other side for 2 minutes, or until the bottom is light brown.
6. Spread Nutella and peanut butter on the crepe, and roll up if desired. Serve and enjoy.

*Note: *If you use a frying pan and there seems to be too much batter in the pan, you can drain the excess batter back into the bowl by tilting the pan over the bowl until the excess is removed, then returning the pan to the heat.**

NOTES:

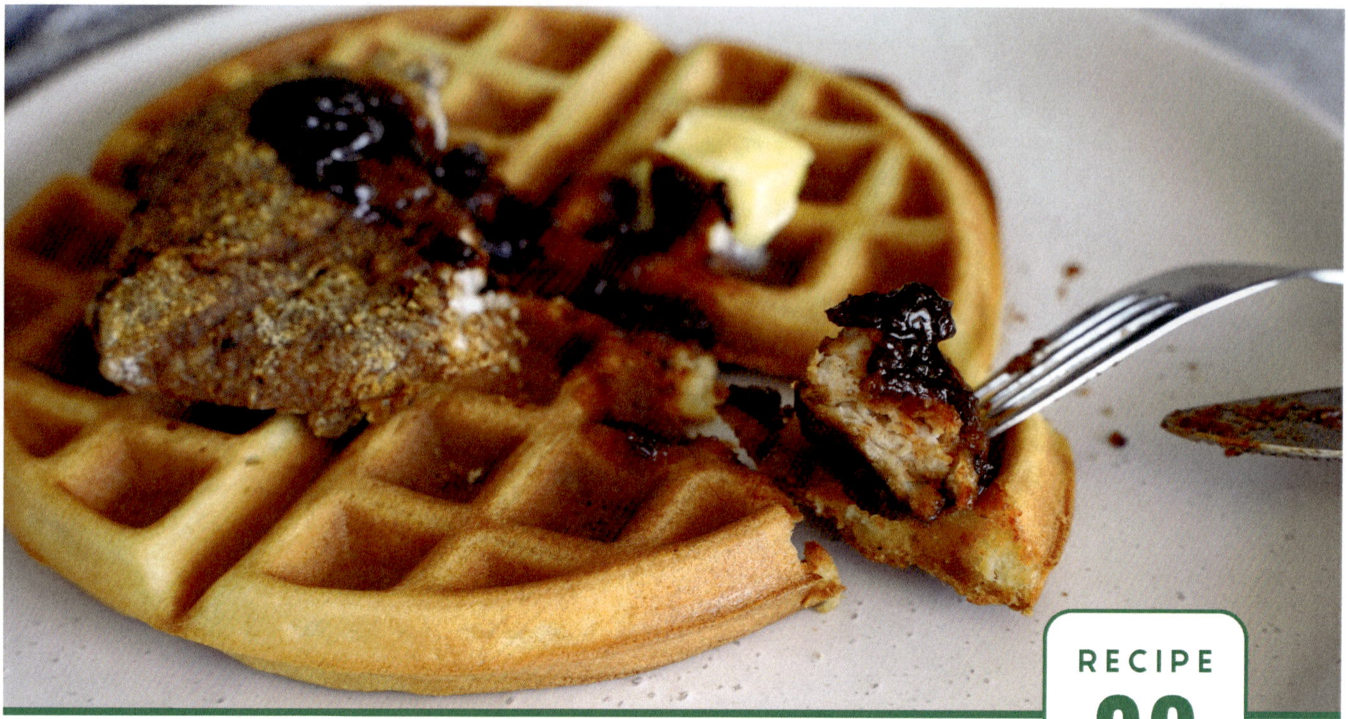

RECIPE 09

OVEN FRIED CHICKEN & WAFFLES

INGREDIENTS

FRIED CHICKEN

2 tablespoons vegetable oil (27.2g)
2 boneless chicken breasts (168g)
1 teaspoon black pepper (2.3g)
1 teaspoon seasoning salt (4.8g)
1 teaspoon lemon pepper (2.8g)
1/2 teaspoon crushed red pepper flakes (1g)
1 teaspoon paprika (6.8g)
1 teaspoon garlic powder (9.7g)
1 teaspoon onion powder (6.9g)
1/2 cup all-purpose flour (62g)
1 teaspoon salt (6g)

INGREDIENTS

HICKORY SWEET CHILI SAUCE

3.5 oz. chipotle peppers in adobo sauce (99.2g), [or combine 3 teaspoons chipotle pepper powder (3g), 3½ tablespoons red wine vinegar (52.2g), and 3½ tablespoons tomato paste - no added salt (56g)]
1/4 cup honey (84.8g)
1/2 teaspoon lemon juice (2.6g)
1/2 teaspoon apple cider (2.3g)
1 teaspoon orange juice (2.5g)
1/2 teaspoon garlic powder (1.6g)
1/2 teaspoon onion powder (1.2g)

INGREDIENTS

WAFFLE INGREDIENTS

2 jumbo eggs (126g)
1¾ cups whole milk (427g)
1/2 cup grapeseed oil (109g)
1½ teaspoons vanilla extract (6.3g)
1¾ cups all-purpose flour (218.8g)
1/4 cup cornstarch (32g)
2 tablespoons granulated sugar (25.2g)
1 tablespoon baking powder (15g)
1/4 teaspoon salt (1.5g)

PREPARATION

CHICKEN:

1. Preheat the oven to 390°F (200°C). Line a baking sheet with baking/parchment paper, or spray a non-stick tray with cooking oil spray.
2. In a medium bowl, add black pepper, seasoning salt, lemon pepper, crushed red pepper flakes, paprika, garlic powder, and onion powder and mix.
3. Use about ¾ of the seasoning mixture above to evenly coat the chicken breasts. Reserve the remaining seasoning mixture for step 4.
4. In a large bowl, combine the flour and remaining seasoning mix; stir well.
5. One by one, evenly coat the chicken breasts in the seasoned flour mixture and place on the prepared baking sheet.
6. Lightly spray each chicken breast with cooking oil spray. (This is optional, but it will help to crisp the chicken.)
7. Bake for 25-30 minutes, or until the chicken is cooked through. The crust should be crispy and golden brown.
8. Remove the chicken from the baking sheet and set aside on a plate until the waffle is ready.

HONEY-CHIPOTLE SAUCE:

1. While chicken cooks, prepare sauce.
2. Place all the ingredients for the sauce in a small saucepan and cook on low heat. Stir continuously until the mixture is smooth.
3. If too sweet, add small amounts of chipotle powder, if too spicy add small amounts of honey to taste.
4. Remove the sauce from the heat, when the chicken and waffles are complete drizzle sauce onto, serve and enjoy.

WAFFLE INSTRUCTIONS:

1. Preheat a waffle iron. Whisk together the eggs, whole milk, oil, and vanilla extract in a medium bowl.
2. Add the flour, cornstarch, sugar, baking powder, and salt, and whisk until the batter is just combined. Over-mixing or mixing until smooth will create tough waffles.
3. Spray the waffle iron liberally with cooking spray. Pour the batter into the waffle iron so it just coats the plates. Close and cook until the waffles are golden brown on the outside, and a toothpick inserted in the center comes out clean. Place the finished waffles on a plate, then place the chicken onto the waffles, and then drizzle sauce onto both. Serve and enjoy.

NOTES:

nutrition facts breakfast

Banana Bread French Toast

Nutrition Facts

5 servings per container
Serving size **1 slice (0.0g)**

Amount Per Serving	
Calories	**690**
	% Daily Value*
Total Fat 30g	**38%**
Saturated Fat 14g	**70%**
Trans Fat 0g	
Cholesterol 295mg	**98%**
Sodium 550mg	**24%**
Total Carbohydrate 89g	**32%**
Dietary Fiber 4g	**14%**
Total Sugars 43g	
Includes 30g Added Sugars	**60%**
Protein 16g	
Vitamin D 1.5mcg	8%
Calcium 150mg	10%
Iron 3.7mg	20%
Potassium 470mg	10%

* The % Daily Value (DV) tells you how much a nutrient in a serving of food contributes to a daily diet. 2,000 calories a day is used for general nutrition advice.

Hot Chocolate Pancakes

Nutrition Facts

1 serving per container
Serving size **4-inch pancake (0.0g)**

Amount Per Serving	
Calories	**550**
	% Daily Value*
Total Fat 23g	**29%**
Saturated Fat 5g	**25%**
Trans Fat 0g	
Polyunsaturated Fat 5g	
Monounsaturated Fat 12g	
Cholesterol 130mg	**43%**
Sodium 1010mg	**44%**
Total Carbohydrate 73g	**27%**
Dietary Fiber 6g	**21%**
Total Sugars 19g	
Includes 13g Added Sugars	**26%**
Protein 16g	
Vitamin D 0.7mcg	4%
Calcium 180mg	15%
Iron 5mg	30%
Potassium 440mg	10%

* The % Daily Value (DV) tells you how much a nutrient in a serving of food contributes to a daily diet. 2,000 calories a day is used for general nutrition advice.

Overnight Oats - Carrot Cake

Nutrition Facts

1 serving per container
Serving size **1.5 cup (0.0g)**

Amount Per Serving	
Calories	**400**
	% Daily Value*
Total Fat 9g	**12%**
Saturated Fat 3g	**15%**
Trans Fat 0g	
Polyunsaturated Fat 1g	
Monounsaturated Fat 1.5g	
Cholesterol 15mg	**5%**
Sodium 120mg	**5%**
Total Carbohydrate 68g	**25%**
Dietary Fiber 9g	**32%**
Total Sugars 36g	
Includes 0g Added Sugars	**0%**
Protein 16g	
Vitamin D 0.1mcg	0%
Calcium 280mg	20%
Iron 2.6mg	15%
Potassium 850mg	20%

* The % Daily Value (DV) tells you how much a nutrient in a serving of food contributes to a daily diet. 2,000 calories a day is used for general nutrition advice.

Overnight Oats - Peachy Clean

Nutrition Facts

1 serving per container
Serving size **1.5 cups (0.0g)**

Amount Per Serving	
Calories	**460**
	% Daily Value*
Total Fat 11g	**14%**
Saturated Fat 4g	**20%**
Trans Fat 0g	
Cholesterol 15mg	**5%**
Sodium 160mg	**7%**
Total Carbohydrate 75g	**27%**
Dietary Fiber 12g	**43%**
Total Sugars 45g	
Includes 17g Added Sugars	**34%**
Protein 17g	
Vitamin D 0.1mcg	0%
Calcium 350mg	25%
Iron 3mg	15%
Potassium 900mg	20%

* The % Daily Value (DV) tells you how much a nutrient in a serving of food contributes to a daily diet. 2,000 calories a day is used for general nutrition advice.

Overnight Oats - Chai'd and True

Nutrition Facts

1 serving per container
Serving size **(0.0g)**

Amount Per Serving	
Calories	**400**
	% Daily Value*
Total Fat 13g	**17%**
Saturated Fat 3.5g	**18%**
Trans Fat 0g	
Cholesterol 15mg	**5%**
Sodium 80mg	**3%**
Total Carbohydrate 51g	**19%**
Dietary Fiber 6g	**21%**
Total Sugars 27g	
Includes 17g Added Sugars	**34%**
Protein 17g	
Vitamin D 0.1mcg	0%
Calcium 270mg	20%
Iron 2.1mg	10%
Potassium 530mg	10%

* The % Daily Value (DV) tells you how much a nutrient in a serving of food contributes to a daily diet. 2,000 calories a day is used for general nutrition advice.

Sweet Potato Hash with Sunny-Side Up Egg

Nutrition Facts

1 serving per container
Serving size **2.5 cup (0.0g)**

Amount Per Serving	
Calories	**760**
	% Daily Value*
Total Fat 31g	**40%**
Saturated Fat 9g	**45%**
Trans Fat 0g	
Polyunsaturated Fat 8g	
Monounsaturated Fat 10g	
Cholesterol 275mg	**92%**
Sodium 4210mg	**183%**
Total Carbohydrate 99g	**36%**
Dietary Fiber 16g	**57%**
Total Sugars 19g	
Includes 0g Added Sugars	**0%**
Protein 25g	
Vitamin D 1.3mcg	6%
Calcium 210mg	15%
Iron 10.1mg	60%
Potassium 1820mg	40%

* The % Daily Value (DV) tells you how much a nutrient in a serving of food contributes to a daily diet. 2,000 calories a day is used for general nutrition advice.

nutrition facts breakfast

Easy Omelet with Flair - Bulk Up

Nutrition Facts

1 serving per container
Serving size 2 egg (0.0g)

Amount Per Serving
Calories 710

	% Daily Value*
Total Fat 44g	**56%**
Saturated Fat 20g	**100%**
Trans Fat 1g	
Cholesterol 575mg	**192%**
Sodium 4050mg	**176%**
Total Carbohydrate 33g	**12%**
Dietary Fiber 3g	**11%**
Total Sugars 6g	
Includes 0g Added Sugars	**0%**
Protein 43g	
Vitamin D 3.3mcg	15%
Calcium 510mg	40%
Iron 5.4mg	30%
Potassium 690mg	15%

* The % Daily Value (DV) tells you how much a nutrient in a serving of food contributes to a daily diet. 2,000 calories a day is used for general nutrition advice.

Easy Omelet with Flair - Veggie Lover

Nutrition Facts

1 serving per container
Serving size 2 egg (0.0g)

Amount Per Serving
Calories 690

	% Daily Value*
Total Fat 45g	**58%**
Saturated Fat 24g	**120%**
Trans Fat 1g	
Cholesterol 550mg	**183%**
Sodium 1220mg	**53%**
Total Carbohydrate 29g	**11%**
Dietary Fiber 7g	**25%**
Total Sugars 14g	
Includes 0g Added Sugars	**0%**
Protein 44g	
Vitamin D 3.1mcg	15%
Calcium 890mg	70%
Iron 4.1mg	25%
Potassium 940mg	20%

* The % Daily Value (DV) tells you how much a nutrient in a serving of food contributes to a daily diet. 2,000 calories a day is used for general nutrition advice.

Easy Omelet with Flair - Southwest

Nutrition Facts

1 serving per container
Serving size 2 egg (0.0g)

Amount Per Serving
Calories 680

	% Daily Value*
Total Fat 51g	**65%**
Saturated Fat 20g	**100%**
Trans Fat 1g	
Polyunsaturated Fat 6g	
Monounsaturated Fat 22g	
Cholesterol 535mg	**178%**
Sodium 910mg	**40%**
Total Carbohydrate 24g	**9%**
Dietary Fiber 11g	**39%**
Total Sugars 8g	
Includes 0g Added Sugars	**0%**
Protein 36g	
Vitamin D 2.6mcg	15%
Calcium 610mg	45%
Iron 3.8mg	20%
Potassium 1240mg	25%

* The % Daily Value (DV) tells you how much a nutrient in a serving of food contributes to a daily diet. 2,000 calories a day is used for general nutrition advice.

Reese's Peanut - Butter Crepes

Nutrition Facts

About 3 servings per container
Serving size 1 crepe (0.0g)

Amount Per Serving
Calories 370

	% Daily Value*
Total Fat 18g	**23%**
Saturated Fat 8g	**40%**
Trans Fat 0g	
Cholesterol 180mg	**60%**
Sodium 280mg	**12%**
Total Carbohydrate 39g	**14%**
Dietary Fiber 2g	**7%**
Total Sugars 6g	
Includes 3g Added Sugars	**6%**
Protein 12g	
Vitamin D 0.9mcg	4%
Calcium 90mg	6%
Iron 2.9mg	15%
Potassium 220mg	4%

* The % Daily Value (DV) tells you how much a nutrient in a serving of food contributes to a daily diet. 2,000 calories a day is used for general nutrition advice.

Oven Fried - Chicken & Waffles

Nutrition Facts

2 servings per container
Serving size 1 container

Amount Per Serving
Calories 1430

	% Daily Value*
Total Fat 65g	**83%**
Saturated Fat 28g	**140%**
Trans Fat 0g	
Polyunsaturated Fat 20g	
Monounsaturated Fat 6g	
Cholesterol 230mg	**77%**
Sodium 4540mg	**197%**
Total Carbohydrate 138g	**50%**
Dietary Fiber 12g	**43%**
Total Sugars 22g	
Includes 13g Added Sugars	**26%**
Protein 62g	**124%**
Vitamin D 0.14mcg	0%
Calcium 4940mg	380%
Iron 1.818mg	10%
Potassium 54426mg	1160%

* The % Daily Value (DV) tells you how much a nutrient in a serving of food contributes to a daily diet. 2,000 calories a day is used for general nutrition advice.

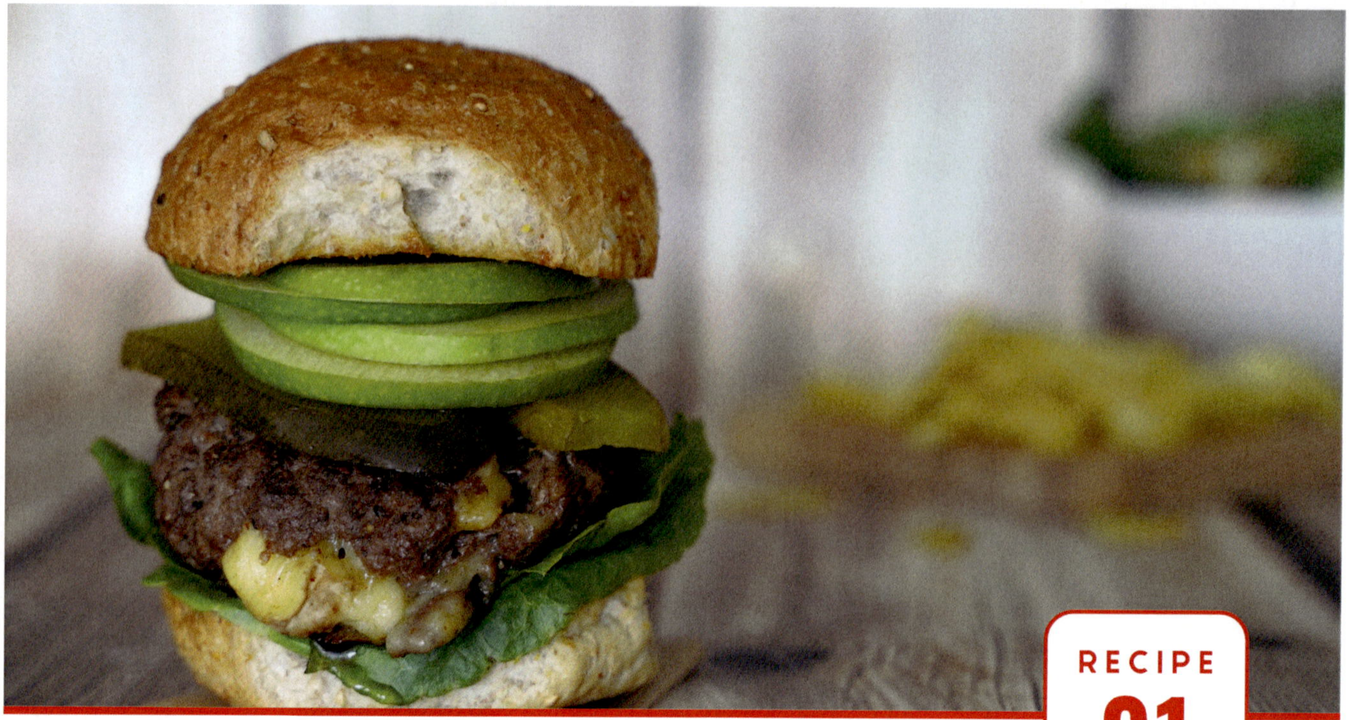

RECIPE 01

THE DOCTOR'S IN

INGREDIENTS

12 oz. 70/30% ground beef (3/4 pound, 340.2g)
1 teaspoon black pepper (2.3g)
1 teaspoon salt (6g)
1 teaspoon lemon pepper (2.8g)
1 teaspoon onion powder (2.4g)
1/2 teaspoon crushed red pepper flakes (1g)
1/8 cup cubed Brie (18g)
1 teaspoon unsalted butter (4.7g)
1 teaspoon honey (6.9g)
4 white hamburger buns (200g)
1/2 cup sliced Granny Smith apple (54.5g)
Garnish - lettuce, sliced tomatoes, pickles

PREPARATION

1. In a large bowl, add the ground beef, black pepper, salt, lemon pepper, onion powder, and crushed red pepper flakes and mix well.
2. Add the Brie pieces to the beef mixture and fold gently to incorporate. Form the mixture into 2 - 6oz—patties, about ¾-inch thick.
3. In a small bowl, combine the butter and honey. Microwave until the butter is melted.
4. Once the burgers are cooked, cut the hamburger buns in half horizontally. Brush the insides of the buns with the honey butter mixture, and toast in a skillet or toaster oven until golden brown.
5. To pan-fry the burgers, heat a large skillet over medium heat. Cook the burgers for 6-10 minutes on each side, or until there is no pink. To grill the burgers, preheat the grill on high heat. Cook the burgers for 6-10 minutes on each side, or until there is no pink, flipping frequently.
6. Place the finished burgers on the toasted buns, top with apple slices, and garnish with desired toppings. Serve and enjoy.

NICK'S NUTRITIONAL NUGGETS

Higher fat content is recommended because it increases the burger's ability to bind when stuffed.

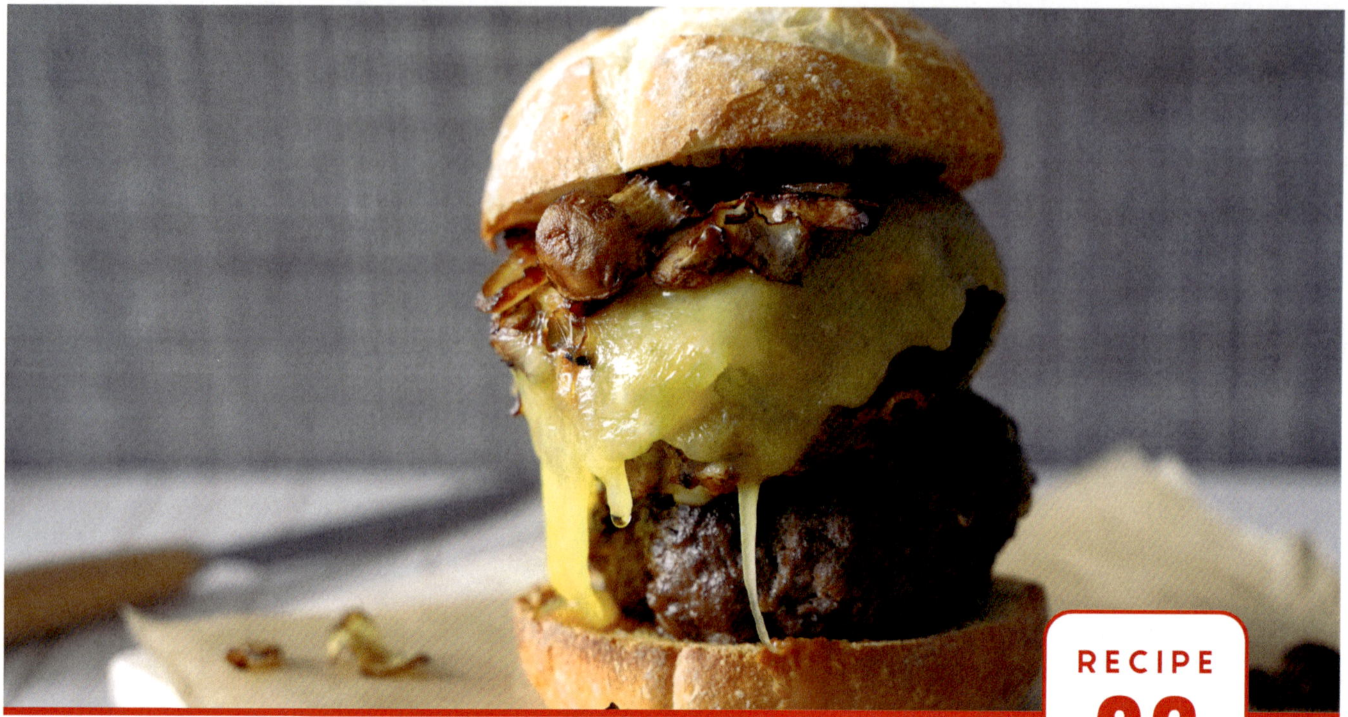

RECIPE 02

IT'S OKAY TO BE CHEESY

INGREDIENTS

12 oz. 70/30% ground beef (3/4 pound, 340.2g)

1 teaspoon black pepper (2.3g)

1 teaspoon salt (6g)

1 teaspoon lemon pepper (2.8g)

1 teaspoon onion powder (2.4g)

1/2 teaspoon crushed red pepper flakes (1g)

1/8 cup crumbled feta cheese (18.8g)

1/8 cup cubed Gouda (19.5g)

2 slices cheddar cheese (56g)

1/4 cup chopped onions (40g)

1/4 cup sliced mushrooms (17.5g)

1/2 tablespoon Worcestershire sauce (8.5g)

1 teaspoon unsalted butter (4.7g)

1 teaspoon honey (6.9g)

4 white hamburger buns (200g)

PREPARATION

1. In a large bowl, add ground beef, black pepper, salt, lemon pepper, onion powder, and crushed red pepper flakes and mix well.
2. Add the feta and Gouda to the beef mixture and fold gently to incorporate. Form the beef mixture into 2 6-ounce patties, about ¾-inch thick.
3. To pan-fry, heat a large skillet over medium heat. Cook the burgers for 6-10 minutes on each side, or until there is no pink, flipping regularly. To grill the burgers, preheat the grill on high heat. Cook the burgers for 6-10 minutes on each side, or until there is no pink, flipping regularly.
4. While the burgers are cooking, set a medium skillet over medium heat and spray with non-stick cooking oil spray. When hot, add the onions, mushrooms, and Worcestershire sauce. Cook for 10 minutes, stirring often, until soft.
5. In a small bowl, combine the butter and honey. Microwave until the butter is melted.
6. Once the burgers are cooked, cut the hamburger buns in half horizontally. Brush the insides of the buns with the honey butter mixture, and toast in a skillet or toaster oven until golden brown.
7. Transfer the burgers to the toasted buns, and top each burger with a slice of cheddar cheese and desired garnish. Serve and enjoy.

NICK'S NUTRITIONAL NUGGETS

Higher fat content is recommended because it increases the burger's ability to bind when stuffed.

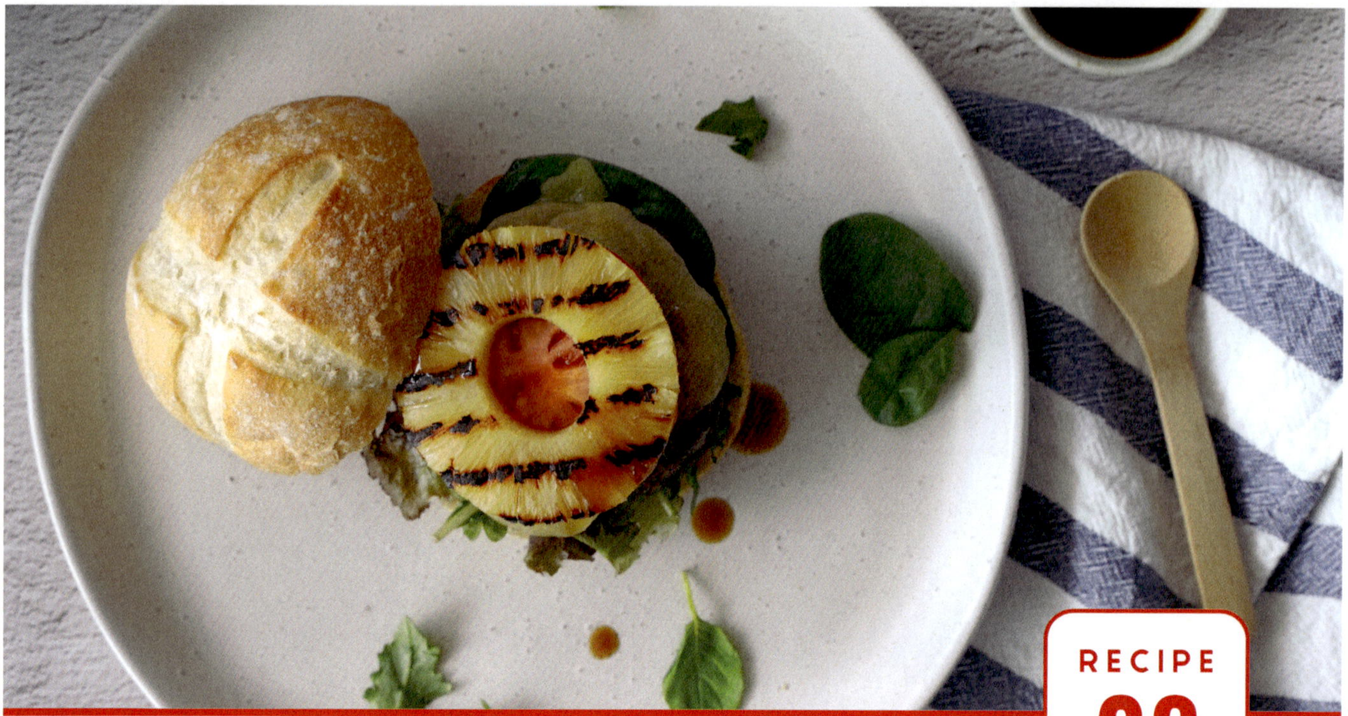

RECIPE 03

THE LUAU

INGREDIENTS

12 oz. 70/30% ground beef (3/4 pound, 340.2g)
1 teaspoon black pepper (2.3g)
1 teaspoon salt (6g)
1 teaspoon lemon pepper (2.8g)
1 teaspoon onion powder (2.4g)
1/2 teaspoon crushed red pepper flakes (1g)
2 slices pineapple (332g)
1 teaspoon unsalted butter (4.7g)
1 teaspoon honey (6.9g)
2 white hamburger buns (200g)
2 slices Pepper Jack cheese (42g)
1 tablespoon reduced-sodium teriyaki sauce (1/2 oz., 14.2g)

PREPARATION

1. In a large bowl, the add ground beef, black pepper, salt, lemon pepper, onion powder, and crushed red pepper flakes and mix well.
2. Form the beef mixture into 2 - 6oz—patties, about ¾-inch thick.
3. To pan-fry the burgers, heat a large skillet over medium heat. Cook the burgers for 6-10 minutes on each side, or until there is no pink. To grill the burgers, preheat the grill on high heat. Cook the burgers for 6-10 minutes on each side, or until there is no pink, flipping regularly.
4. While the burgers are cooking, place the pineapple slices on the grill; if using a skillet, place the pineapple slices in the skillet after the burgers have been completely cooked and removed from the skillet. Cook for 3-5 minutes, flipping halfway through.
5. In a small bowl, combine the butter and honey. Microwave until the butter is melted.
6. Once the burgers are cooked, cut the hamburger buns in half horizontally. Brush the insides of the buns with the honey butter mixture, and toast in a skillet or toaster oven until golden brown.
7. Transfer the burgers to the toasted buns and top each with a slice of Pepper Jack cheese, followed by a pineapple ring and ½ a tablespoon of teriyaki sauce on each burger. Finish with any desired garnish, serve and enjoy.

NICK'S NUTRITIONAL NUGGETS

Higher fat content is recommended because it increases the burger's ability to bind when stuffed.

LUNCH RECIPES

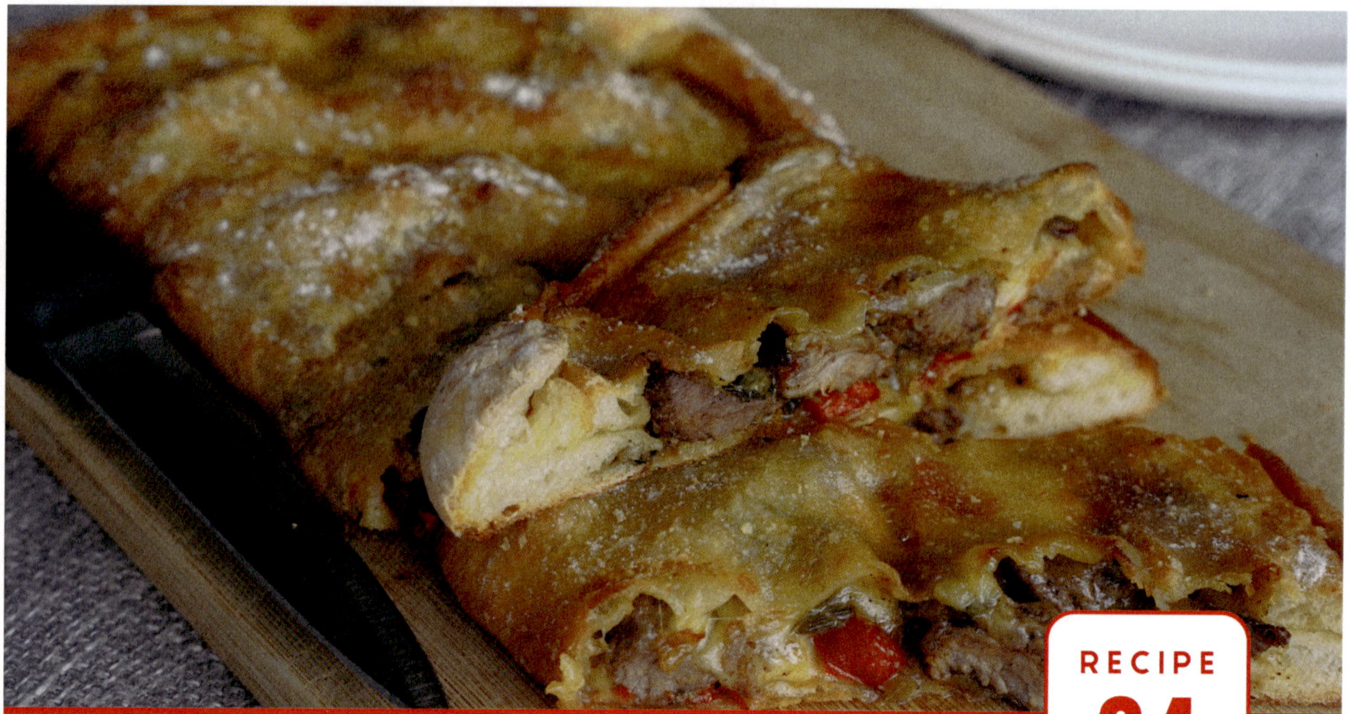

RECIPE 04

PHILLY CHEESESTEAK CALZONE

INGREDIENTS

1 can Pillsbury Classic Pizza Crust (13.8 oz., 391.2g)
6 oz. sliced thin and chopped steak (1/4 pound, 170.1g)
1 teaspoon lemon pepper (2.8g)
1 teaspoon salt (6g)
1 teaspoon black pepper (2.3g)
1 teaspoon onion powder (2.4g)
1/4 teaspoon crushed red pepper flakes (0.5g)
1/4 cup chopped spinach (7.5g)
1/4 cup chopped bell pepper (37.3g)
1/4 cup thinly sliced green onion (17.8g)
1½ cups shredded mozzarella cheese (168g)
1 tablespoon unsalted butter - melted (14.2g)

PREPARATION

1. Preheat the oven to 350°F (175°C).
2. Roll out the pizza crust dough on a lightly floured surface. Gently shape into a 16x10-inch rectangle. Transfer to a lightly greased cookie sheet.
3. Season the steak with lemon pepper, salt, pepper, onion powder, and crushed red pepper flakes.
4. Lightly grease a large skillet and set over medium heat. Once hot, add the steak and cook for 10-15 minutes, or until just cooked through.
5. Arrange the meat, vegetables, and cheese down half of the dough lengthwise.
6. Fold the dough over the filling and tuck the loose ends under the filled dough. Brush the top of the dough with butter.
7. Make 4-5 cuts in the top of the dough, spaced 2-3 inches apart.
8. Bake for 30-40 minutes or until golden brown and the edges are flaky. Allow to cool for 10 minutes before serving.

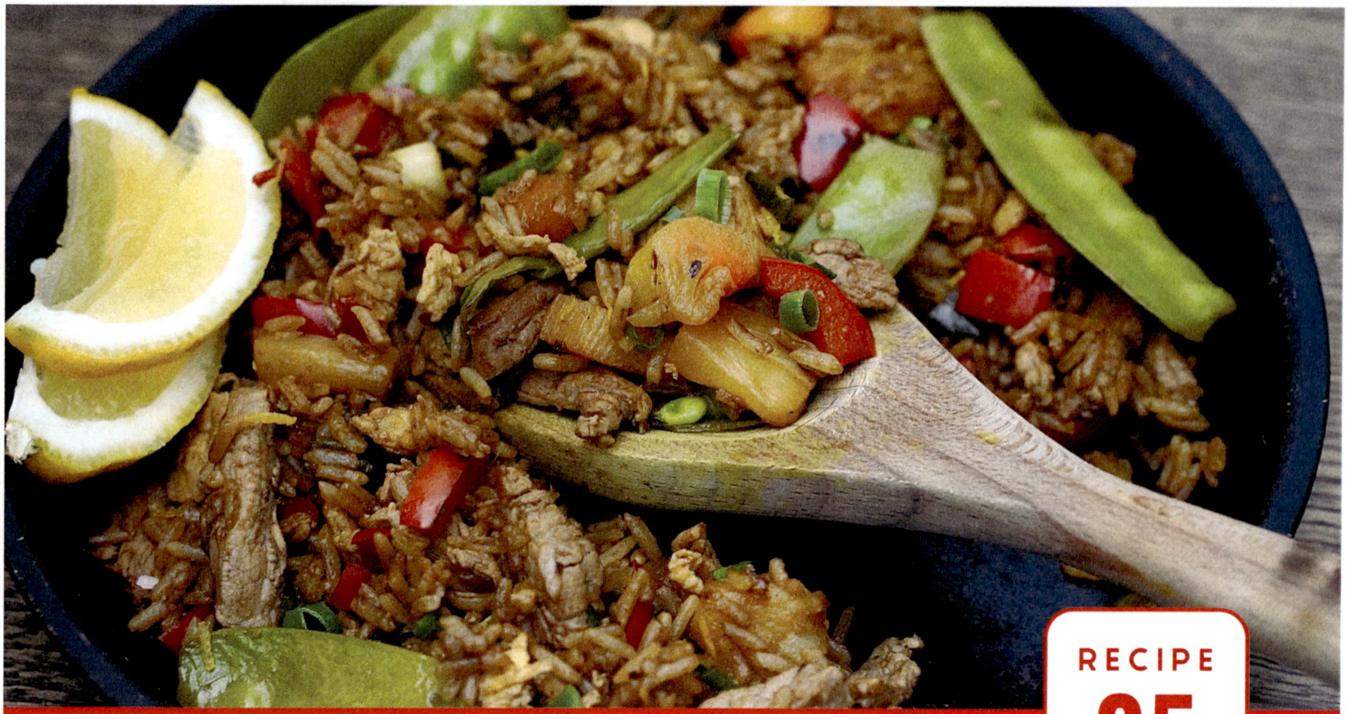

RECIPE 05

TROPICAL PORK FRIED RICE

INGREDIENTS

1 cup uncooked long grain white rice (3 cups cooked (fresh or day-old rice) (158g)
2 cups water (474g)
6 oz. chopped lean pork (170g)
1/4 teaspoon salt (1.5g)
1/2 teaspoon black pepper (1.2g)
1/2 teaspoon all-purpose seasoning (0.6g)
3 teaspoons extra-virgin olive oil (14g)
2 large eggs (126g)
1½ cups chopped pineapple (247.5g)
1 chopped large red pepper (164g)
3/4 cup chopped green onions (53.3g)
1¼ cups snow peas (78.8g)
1 teaspoon minced garlic –(5g)
1/4 cup low-sodium soy sauce (63.8g)
1/2 cup chopped mango (82.5g)
1/2 tablespoon grated lemon zest (3g)

PREPARATION

1. If using fresh rice, continue to step 3
2. If using one-day-old rice, skip to step 8
3. In a fine strainer, rinse rice under cold water until the water runs clear.
4. In a medium saucepan over medium heat, bring the water to a boil. Add rice and a pinch of salt.
5. Bring to a low boil, then lower heat, cover the saucepan and cook covered for 18 minutes, or until the rice is tender and all the water is absorbed.
6. Turn off the heat, strain the rice to remove excess liquid, if any, and then set aside for 5 minutes. Fluff with a fork, and then set aside for later use.
7. To quickly cool the rice, spread it across a parchment-lined rimmed baking sheet and let it cool in the fridge for 30 minutes or in the freezer for 10-15 minutes until it is thoroughly chilled. If using the freezer, make sure the rice does not freeze.
8. Heat a large wok, cast-iron skillet, or non-stick frying pan over medium-high heat. Season the pork with salt, pepper, and all-purpose seasoning and cook for 10-15 minutes, or until juices run clear. Transfer pork to a large bowl and set aside.
9. Wipe out the pan if necessary, with a paper towel (be careful, it's hot!).
10. Add a teaspoon of oil to the skillet, then add eggs, and cook, stirring often for 30 seconds to 1 minute or until eggs are scrambled and lightly set. Transfer the eggs into the bowl with the pork.
11. Wipe out the pan again, if necessary, with a paper towel (be careful, it's hot!).
12. Add a teaspoon of oil to the skillet, and then add the chopped pineapple and red pepper. Cook, stirring constantly, for 2-4 minutes or until the liquid has evaporated and the pineapple is caramelized on the edges. Add the green onion, snow peas, and garlic. Cook until fragrant, stirring constantly, for about 30 seconds.
13. Remove the rice from the refrigerator. Add a teaspoon of oil to the skillet and combine the rice, egg, pork mixture, soy sauce, mangos, and lemon zest. Cook for 3-5 minutes, stirring often to break apart the egg and rice. When all the ingredients are thoroughly heated, transfer to a serving dish, and enjoy.

NICK'S NUTRITIONAL NUGGETS

For most types of rice, use a ratio of 1 cup rice to 2 cups water, which you can scale up or down.

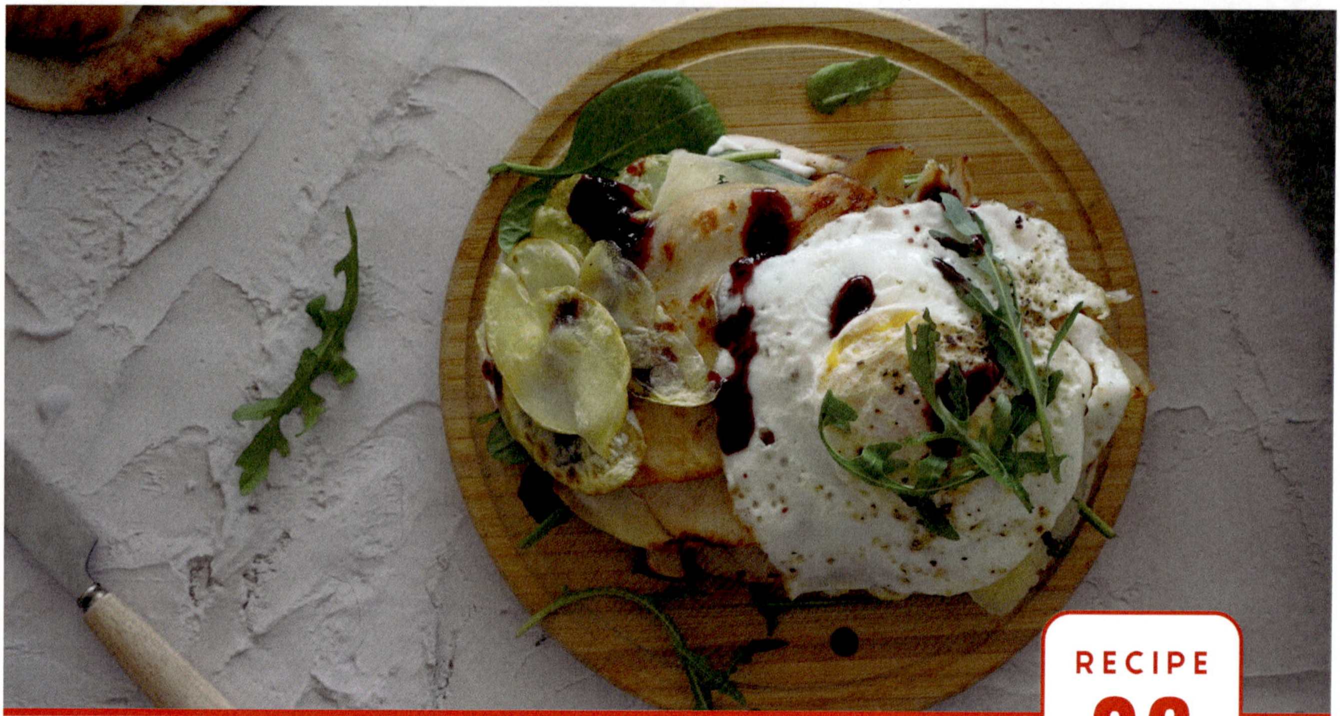

RECIPE 06

RISE AND SHINE TURKEY SANDWICH

INGREDIENTS

SANDWICH

- 2¼ tablespoons extra-virgin olive oil (31.5g)
- 1 jumbo egg (63g)
- Pinch of salt
- Pinch of black pepper
- 1/2 Russet potato – thinly sliced (85g)
- 4 oz. sliced turkey (1/4 pound, 113.4g)
- 1 slice sharp cheddar (19g)
- 1 tablespoon Greek yogurt (1/2 oz., 14.2g)
- 1 whole wheat pita (64g)
- 1/2 cup spinach (15g)
- 2 tomato slices (30g)

INGREDIENTS

CRANBERRY POMEGRANATE SAUCE

- 1 cup fresh cranberries (100g), [or 1 cup fresh cherries – unpitted (154g)]
- 1/4 cup granulated sugar (50g)
- 1/4 cup water (59.3g)
- 1 tablespoon lemon zest (6g)
- 2 tablespoons pomegranate juice (1 oz., 31.4g)
- 1/2 teaspoon cinnamon (1.3g)
- 1/4 teaspoon salt (1.5g)

PREPARATION

SANDWICH INSTRUCTIONS:

1. Set a medium non-stick skillet over medium heat and add 1 teaspoon extra-virgin olive oil. Crack the egg into a skillet and cook for 3 minutes, until white is set—season with a pinch of salt and pepper. Flip and cook the other side, being careful not to break the yolk, for 3-5 minutes or until the yolk is completely set. Season this side with another pinch of salt and pepper. Remove the egg from the skillet and place it on a plate.
2. Bring a medium pot filled halfway with water to a boil. Once the water is boiling, add the sliced potatoes. Reduce the heat to medium-high and cook for 7-10 minutes, or until the potatoes are soft. Drain the potatoes well. Make the cranberry/cherry sauce in accordance with the instructions provided below.
3. Set a medium non-stick skillet over medium heat and add 2 tablespoons of extra-virgin olive oil. Add the sliced potatoes and cook for 5-7 minutes or until golden brown with crisp edges. Remove the potatoes from the skillet and place on a plate.
4. In the same skillet, over medium heat, add the turkey and sear for 3 minutes on each side. Add the sharp cheddar, if you would like melted cheese.
5. Spread the Greek yogurt and 1 tablespoon of cranberry pomegranate sauce on top of the pita and add the spinach, potatoes, cheese (if not already melted on the turkey) tomato slices, turkey, and egg. Serve immediately.

CRANBERRY POMEGRANATE SAUCE:

1. Rinse out the pot used for the potatoes and add the cranberries or cherries, sugar, water, lemon zest, pomegranate juice, cinnamon, and salt. Bring the mixture to a boil over medium heat. Stir well and reduce the heat to low.
2. Allow cranberries to simmer for 15 minutes or cherries 30 minutes to simmer, occasionally stirring, until the cranberries have popped or cherries have liquefied. Remove from the heat and let cool slightly before serving.

NICK'S NUTRITIONAL NUGGETS

Zest is the colorful portion of the peel or rind. Äîboth is the colorful outer portion and the bitter white pith that lies right beneath. Zest has the bright flavor of the fruit. The colorful zest adds the bright acidic flavor of the fruit.

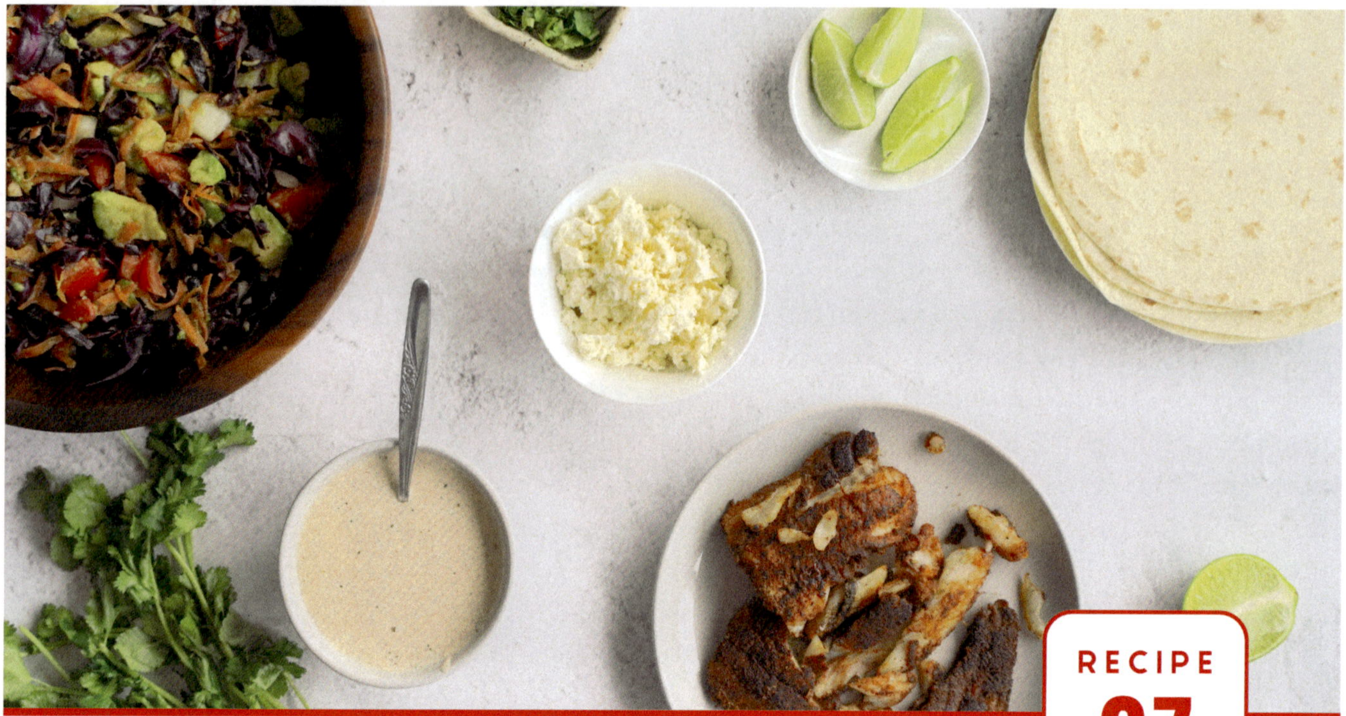

RECIPE 07

COD TACOS WITH CHIPOTLE RANCH

INGREDIENTS

CHIPOTLE RANCH

1/2 cup mayonnaise (110g)

1/2 cup Greek yogurt (113.4g)

1/2 cup whole milk (122g)

1/2 packet Hidden Valley Ranch seasoning (1/2 oz., 14.2g)

3/4 teaspoons chipotle seasoning (0.75g)

1/2 tablespoon lime juice (about 1/ lime, 1/ oz., 7.7g)

INGREDIENTS

COLE SLAW

2 cups shredded red cabbage (about 1/2 small head, 178g)

1/2 teaspoon kosher salt (3g)

1/2 tablespoon olive oil (6.8g)

1 tablespoon freshly squeezed lime juice (15.4g)

1 teaspoon minced garlic (5g)

1/4 teaspoon black pepper (0.5g)

1/2 cup chopped tomato (90g)

1/4 cup chopped onion (40g)

1 avocado - pitted, peeled, and chopped (201g)

1 grated medium carrot (1/2 cup, 55g)

1/4 cup chopped fresh cilantro (4g)

INGREDIENTS

COD

- 1 teaspoon ground cumin (0.5g)
- 1 teaspoon paprika (6.8g)
- 1 teaspoon onion powder (2.4g)
- 1 teaspoon garlic powder (3.1g)
- 1 teaspoon kosher salt (6g)
- 1 teaspoon black pepper (2.9g)
- 2 - 3 oz. cod fillets (170g)
- 1½ tablespoon olive oil - for tortillas (20.3g)
- 2 white tortillas (60g)
- 1 cup crumbled feta cheese (150g)
- 1/4 cup cilantro leaves (4g)
- Lime wedges (33.5g)

PREPARATION

CHIPOTLE RANCH:

1. Combine mayonnaise, Greek yogurt, milk, Ranch Seasoning packet, chipotle seasoning, and lime juice in a medium bowl and whisk well.
2. Cover and chill for 30 minutes to allow the sauce to thicken.

COLE SLAW:

1. Place the shredded cabbage in a colander set over a bowl, and sprinkle with a pinch of kosher salt. Squeeze cabbage to drain excess liquid and begin wilting. Set aside to continue draining for about 15 minutes.
2. Place the olive oil, lime juice, minced garlic, kosher salt, and black pepper in a large bowl and whisk to combine.
3. Using your hands, squeeze the cabbage of its excess liquid.
4. Mix the cabbage, chopped tomatoes, onions, avocado, grated carrots, and cilantro in the olive oil and seasoning mixture. Set aside until ready to use.

COD:

1. Mix the cumin, paprika, onion powder, garlic powder, kosher salt, and black pepper in a small bowl. Season the cod fillets well on all sides with the spice mix.
2. Set a medium skillet over medium-high heat and add 1/2 tablespoon of olive oil. Warm the tortillas on both sides until lightly browned, about 30 seconds per side, remove and set aside.
3. In the same skillet, heat 1 tablespoon of oil. When hot, add the cod and cook for 4-5 minutes on each side, or until flaky and cooked through.
4. Top each tortilla with a piece of cod, coleslaw mixture, feta cheese, cilantro leaves, and chipotle ranch. Serve with lime wedges and enjoy.

nutrition facts lunch

Burgers with Flair - The Doctors In

Nutrition Facts

1 serving per container
Serving size **2 burger (0.0g)**

Amount Per Serving	
Calories	**1860**
	% Daily Value*
Total Fat 117g	**150%**
Saturated Fat 46g	**230%**
Trans Fat 7g	
Cholesterol 295mg	**98%**
Sodium 4120mg	**179%**
Total Carbohydrate 122g	**44%**
Dietary Fiber 7g	**25%**
Total Sugars 24g	
Includes 6g Added Sugars	**12%**
Protein 70g	
Vitamin D 0.3mcg	2%
Calcium 680mg	50%
Iron 12.2mg	70%
Potassium 1000mg	20%

* The % Daily Value (DV) tells you how much a nutrient in a serving of food contributes to a daily diet. 2,000 calories a day is used for general nutrition advice.

Burgers with Flair - It's Okay to be Cheesy

Nutrition Facts

1 serving per container
Serving size **2 burger (0.0g)**

Amount Per Serving	
Calories	**2130**
	% Daily Value*
Total Fat 140g	**179%**
Saturated Fat 59g	**295%**
Trans Fat 7g	
Cholesterol 370mg	**123%**
Sodium 4620mg	**201%**
Total Carbohydrate 122g	**44%**
Dietary Fiber 6g	**21%**
Total Sugars 22g	
Includes 6g Added Sugars	**12%**
Protein 87g	
Vitamin D 0.8mcg	4%
Calcium 1270mg	100%
Iron 12.6mg	70%
Potassium 1060mg	25%

* The % Daily Value (DV) tells you how much a nutrient in a serving of food contributes to a daily diet. 2,000 calories a day is used for general nutrition advice.

Burgers with Flair - The Lava

Nutrition Facts

1 serving per container
Serving size **2 burger (0.0g)**

Amount Per Serving	
Calories	**2080**
	% Daily Value*
Total Fat 124g	**159%**
Saturated Fat 49g	**245%**
Trans Fat 6g	
Cholesterol 315mg	**105%**
Sodium 4330mg	**188%**
Total Carbohydrate 159g	**58%**
Dietary Fiber 10g	**36%**
Total Sugars 53g	
Includes 7g Added Sugars	**14%**
Protein 78g	
Vitamin D 0.3mcg	2%
Calcium 970mg	70%
Iron 12.9mg	70%
Potassium 1190mg	25%

* The % Daily Value (DV) tells you how much a nutrient in a serving of food contributes to a daily diet. 2,000 calories a day is used for general nutrition advice.

Philly Cheesesteak Calzone

Nutrition Facts

4 servings per container
Serving size **1 Calzone (0.0g)**

Amount Per Serving	
Calories	**460**
	% Daily Value*
Total Fat 18g	**23%**
Saturated Fat 9g	**45%**
Trans Fat 0g	
Cholesterol 70mg	**23%**
Sodium 1520mg	**66%**
Total Carbohydrate 49g	**18%**
Dietary Fiber 2g	**7%**
Total Sugars 7g	
Includes 6g Added Sugars	**12%**
Protein 26g	
Vitamin D 0.2mcg	0%
Calcium 230mg	20%
Iron 3.9mg	20%
Potassium 230mg	4%

* The % Daily Value (DV) tells you how much a nutrient in a serving of food contributes to a daily diet. 2,000 calories a day is used for general nutrition advice.

nutrition facts lunch

Tropical Pork Fried Rice

Nutrition Facts

About 3 servings per container

Serving size	**1 (0.0g)**
Amount Per Serving	
Calories	**330**
	% Daily Value*
Total Fat 10g	**13%**
Saturated Fat 2.5g	**13%**
Trans Fat 0g	
Cholesterol 190mg	**63%**
Sodium 1110mg	**48%**
Total Carbohydrate 38g	**14%**
Dietary Fiber 4g	**14%**
Total Sugars 16g	
Includes 0g Added Sugars	**0%**
Protein 23g	
Vitamin D 1mcg	4%
Calcium 90mg	6%
Iron 3.4mg	20%
Potassium 660mg	15%

* The % Daily Value (DV) tells you how much a nutrient in a serving of food contributes to a daily diet. 2,000 calories a day is used for general nutrition advice.

Rise and Shine Turkey Sandwich

Nutrition Facts

1 serving per container

Serving size	**1 sandwhich (0.0g)**
Amount Per Serving	
Calories	**1060**
	% Daily Value*
Total Fat 48g	**62%**
Saturated Fat 11g	**55%**
Trans Fat 0g	
Cholesterol 300mg	**100%**
Sodium 2200mg	**96%**
Total Carbohydrate 125g	**45%**
Dietary Fiber 11g	**39%**
Total Sugars 64g	
Includes 50g Added Sugars	**100%**
Protein 43g	
Vitamin D 1.5mcg	8%
Calcium 260mg	20%
Iron 5.6mg	30%
Potassium 1200mg	25%

* The % Daily Value (DV) tells you how much a nutrient in a serving of food contributes to a daily diet. 2,000 calories a day is used for general nutrition advice.

Cod Tacos with Chipotle Ranch

Nutrition Facts

1 serving per container

Serving size	**I taco (0.0g)**
Amount Per Serving	
Calories	**710**
	% Daily Value*
Total Fat 47g	**60%**
Saturated Fat 16g	**80%**
Trans Fat 0.5g	
Cholesterol 105mg	**35%**
Sodium 2880mg	**125%**
Total Carbohydrate 48g	**17%**
Dietary Fiber 14g	**50%**
Total Sugars 11g	
Includes 0g Added Sugars	**0%**
Protein 32g	
Vitamin D 0.7mcg	4%
Calcium 520mg	40%
Iron 4.6mg	25%
Potassium 1410mg	30%

* The % Daily Value (DV) tells you how much a nutrient in a serving of food contributes to a daily diet. 2,000 calories a day is used for general nutrition advice.

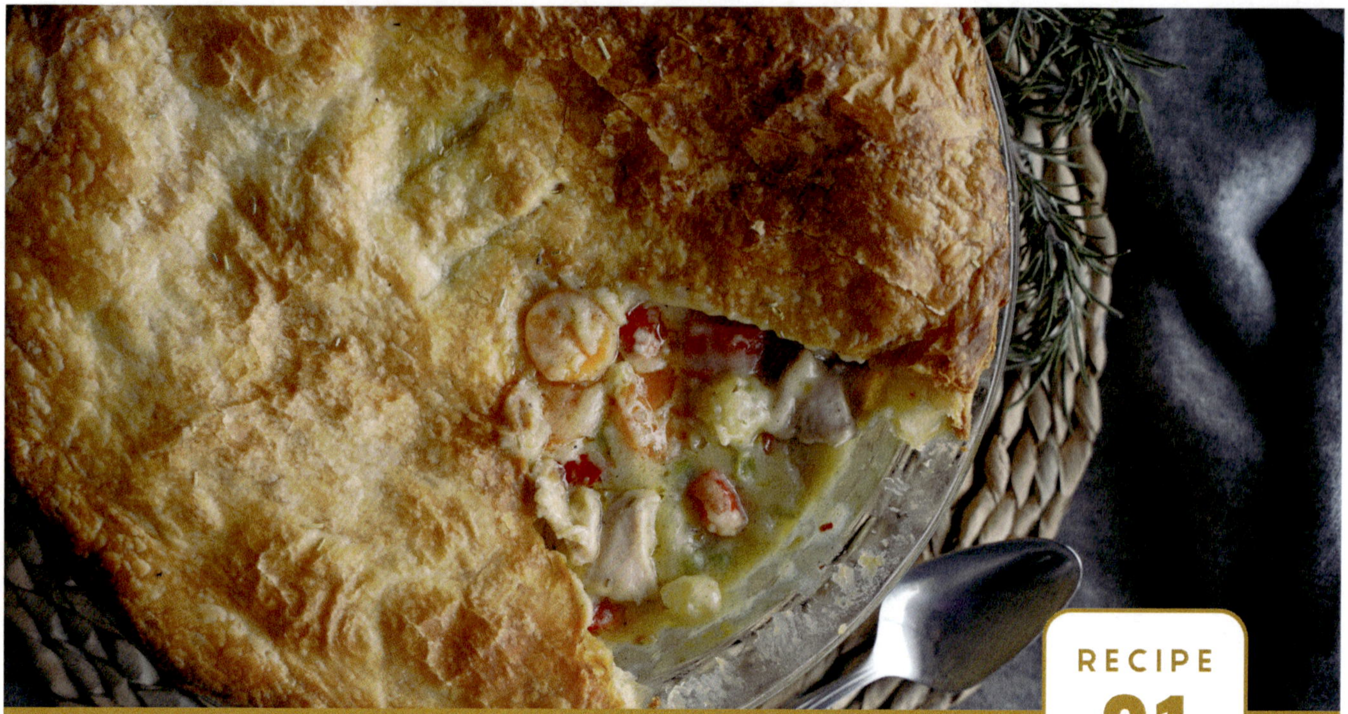

RECIPE 01

ROSEMARY GRAVY CHICKEN POT PIE

INGREDIENTS

- 4 cups shredded or diced chicken (603.3g)
- 1/2 teaspoon seasoning salt (2.4g)
- 1/2 teaspoon lemon pepper (1.4g)
- 1/4 teaspoon crushed red pepper flakes (0.5g)
- 1/2 teaspoon garlic powder (1.6g)
- 1/2 teaspoon onion powder (1.2g)
- 1 teaspoon black pepper (2.3g)
- 2 cups peeled and diced potatoes (312g)
- 1¾ cups sliced carrots (213.5g)
- 1 cup cubed butter (227g)
- 2/3 cup chopped onion (120g)
- 1 cup all-purpose flour (125g)
- 1/2 teaspoon salt (3g)
- 1 teaspoon dried thyme (1g)
- 2½ cups low sodium chicken broth (720g)
- 1½ cups whole milk (366g)
- 2 sprigs chopped rosemary (1 tablespoon, 3.4g)
- 1 cup frozen peas (134g)
- 1 cup diced red bell peppers (149g)
- 4 sheets refrigerated pie crust (916g)

PREPARATION

1. Season the chicken with seasoning salt, lemon pepper, crushed red pepper flakes, garlic powder, onion powder, and 1/4 teaspoon of black pepper. Spray a large skillet with non-stick cooking spray. Place over medium heat, cook the chicken for 15 -20 minutes, or until no pink is present. Set aside to cool.
2. Preheat the oven to 425°F (220°C).
3. In a large saucepan, combine all the potatoes and carrots, and add enough water to cover.
4. Bring the water to a boil, then reduce the heat to medium-low. Cook, covered, for 8-10 minutes, or until crisp-tender. Drain the water.
5. In a large skillet, heat the butter over medium-high heat. Add the onion and cook, stirring occasionally, until tender. Stir in flour and remaining seasonings: salt, dried thyme, and 3/4 teaspoon of black pepper, and mix until blended.
6. Gradually stir in the broth, milk, and chopped rosemary, stirring constantly to prevent lumps forming. Bring to a boil and cook, constantly stirring, for 2 minutes or until thickened. Stir in the chicken, peas, bell pepper, potato/carrot mixture, and remove from the heat. Allow to cool before proceeding to the next step.
7. Unroll a pie crust into each of two 9-inch pie plates. Trim to fit evenly within the rims.
8. Divide the chicken filling between the crusts. Unroll the remaining crusts and place over the filling. Trim, seal, and flute the edges. Cut a few slits in the tops to allow steam to escape.
9. Bake for 35-40 minutes, or until the crust is lightly browned. Let stand for 15 minutes before cutting and serving.
10. Freezing Instructions: Cover the unbaked pies with aluminum foil or plastic wrap and freeze. To use, remove from the freezer 30 minutes before baking (do not thaw).
11. To bake the frozen pies, preheat the oven to 425° (220°C). Place the pies on baking sheets and cover the edges loosely with foil. Bake for 30 minutes, reduce oven temperature to 350°F (175°C), and bake for 70-80 minutes longer, or until the crust is golden brown. Let cool for 15 minutes before cutting and serving.

*Note: *Pre-bake piecrust for 10 minutes, for a crisper crust**

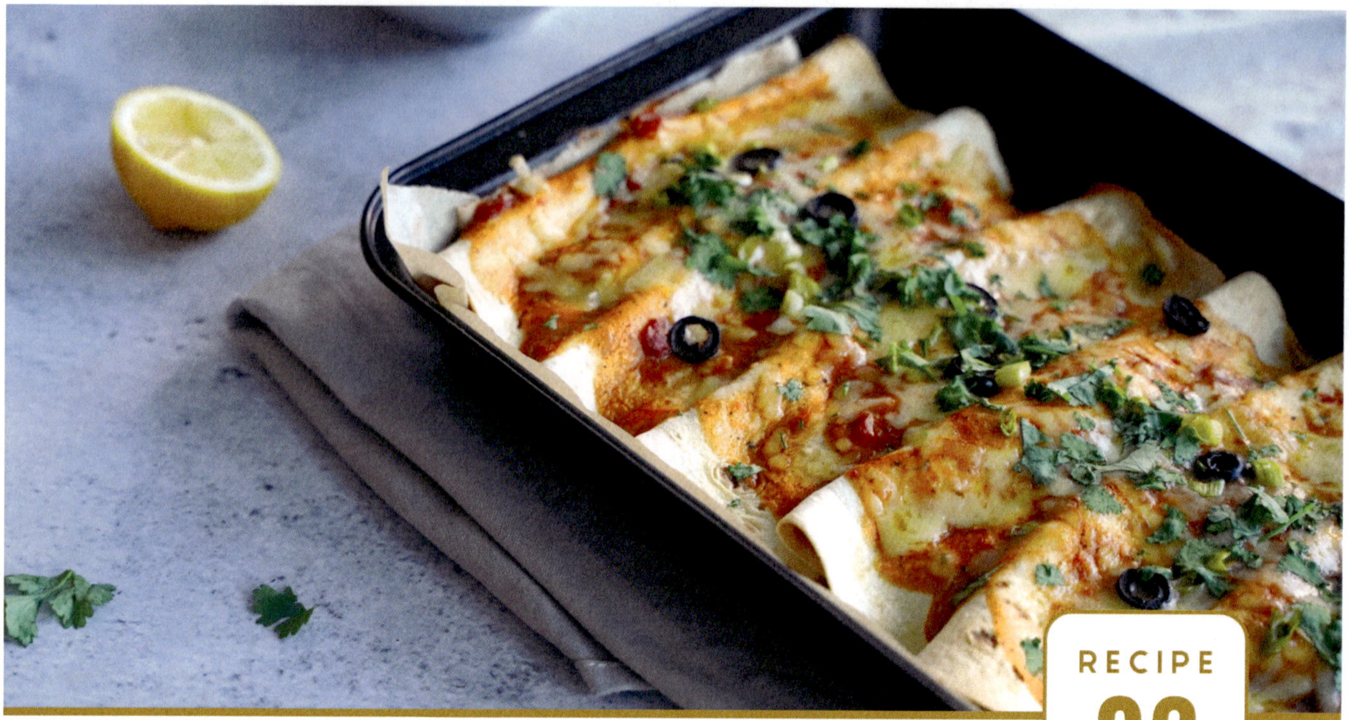

DINNER RECIPES

PINK ENCHILADAS

RECIPE 02

INGREDIENTS

5 oz. Bertolli Alfredo sauce (141.8g)
7 oz. Enchilada sauce (198.5g)
1 cup low-sodium chicken broth (240g)
1/2 teaspoon salt (3g)
1/4 teaspoon black pepper (0.6g)
1/2 pound 80/20% ground beef (226.8g)
1 cup finely chopped yellow onion (87g)
2 tablespoons canola oil (28g)
6 corn tortillas (144g)
4 oz. can diced green chilies (113.4g)
1/2 cup chopped green onions (35.5g)
1/4 cup chopped black olives (56.7g)
1½ cups shredded sharp cheddar cheese (169.5g)
Cilantro, for garnish

PREPARATION

1. In a saucepan over medium-low heat, combine the Alfredo and enchilada sauce. Whisk together and allow to boil for 1 minute.
2. Add the chicken broth, salt, and black pepper, and bring back to a boil.
3. Reduce the heat and simmer while you prepare the other ingredients.
4. While the sauce is simmering, in a large skillet over medium heat, cook the ground beef and onions for 15-17 minutes, or until the meat is browned and the onions are soft. Transfer to a colander and drain the fat.
5. Return the meat and onions to the pan, and then stir to combine. Then turn off the heat and set it aside.
6. In a small skillet over medium heat, heat 1 tablespoon of canola oil for two minutes or until the oil sizzles when a drop of water is added.
7. Line a plate with paper towels. Lightly fry the tortillas in the hot oil just until soft. Do not crisp. When done, transfer to the plate. Repeat until all the tortillas have been fried.
8. Preheat the oven to 350°F (175°C).
9. Spread 1/2 cup of the sauce in the bottom of a 9x13-inch baking dish.
10. One at a time, lay one side of each tortilla into the remaining sauce and set the sauce-soaked tortilla on a plate.
11. Add some of the meat mixture, chilies, green onions, and black olives. Top with a generous portion of shredded cheddar. Roll up the tortilla to contain the filling inside, and place the tortilla, seam side down, in the baking dish.
12. Repeat with the rest of the tortillas and pour the remaining sauce over the top.
13. Top with a generous sprinkling of cheese, chilies, green onions, or olives left over from the filling.
14. Bake the enchiladas for 20 minutes or until bubbly.
15. Remove from the oven, sprinkle chopped cilantro over the top, and serve.

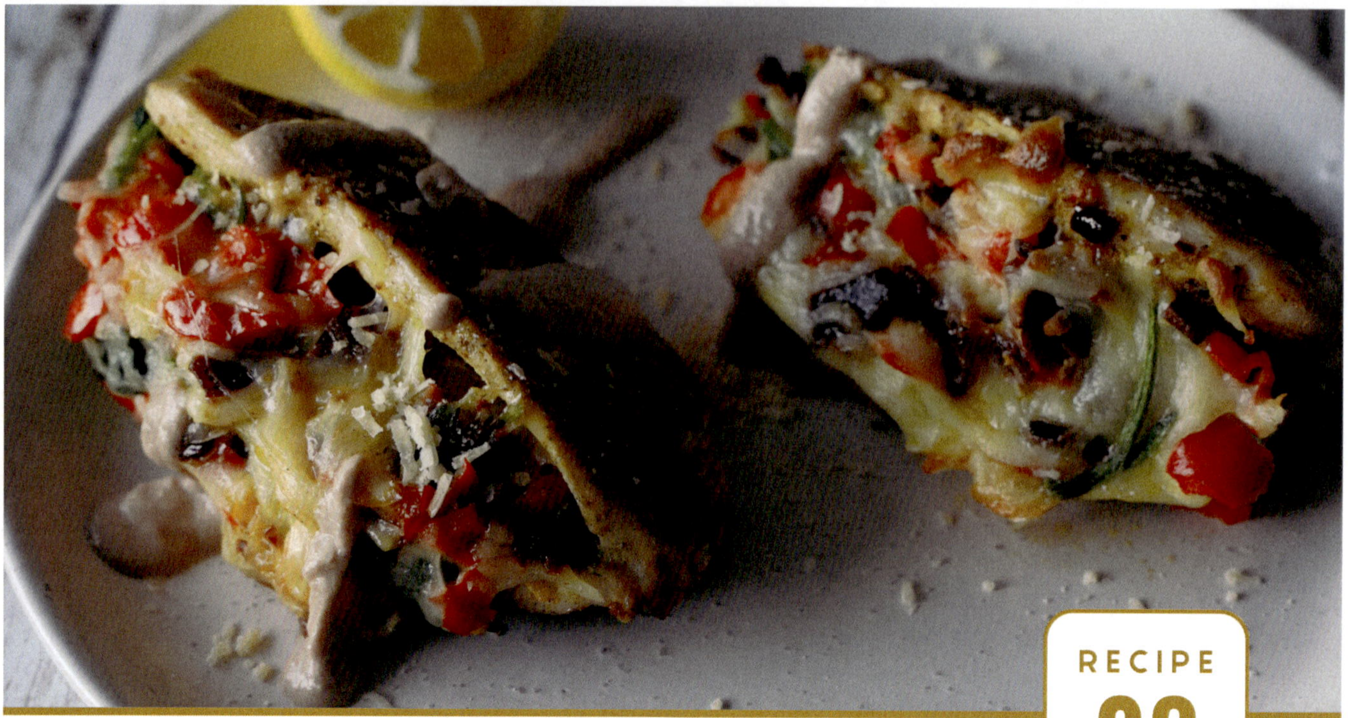

DINNER RECIPES

RECIPE 03

BALSAMIC STUFFED CHICKEN TACO

INGREDIENTS

STUFF CHICKEN TACO

- 2 tablespoons brown sugar - packed (18g)
- 4 slices thick-cut bacon turkey bacon - or favorite bacon (32.4g)
- 2 - 6 oz. chicken breasts (340.2g)
- 1/2 teaspoon poultry seasoning (0.8g)
- 1/2 teaspoon black pepper (1.2g)
- 1/8 teaspoon salt (0.8g)
- 1/2 teaspoon lemon pepper (1.4g)
- 1/4 teaspoon crushed red pepper flakes (0.5g)
- 1/2 teaspoon seasoning salt (2.4g)
- 1/2 teaspoon garlic powder (1.6g)
- 1/2 teaspoon onion powder (1.2g)
- 1 tablespoon extra-virgin olive oil (14g)
- 1/2 cup chopped red bell peppers (75g)
- 2 teaspoons minced garlic (10g)
- 2 cups spinach (60g)
- 1 cup shredded mozzarella cheese (112g)

PREPARATION

STUFF CHICKEN TACO:

1. Preheat oven to 350°F (175°C).
2. Spread the brown sugar on a baking sheet and lay the bacon on it, covering both sides. Bake for 12 minutes, or until golden brown with a strong aroma. Wait until bacon is cooled, crumble it, and set aside.
3. Cut a horizontal slit in the chicken breasts to form a pocket. Season on all sides and inside the pockets with the poultry seasoning, black pepper, salt, lemon pepper, crushed red pepper, seasoning salt, garlic powder, and onion powder.
4. In a large skillet, add half of the olive oil over medium heat and sauté the red peppers and garlic for 10 minutes, or until soft. Remove from skillet and set aside.
5. In the same large skillet, heat the remaining olive oil over medium heat and add the chicken breasts. Cook for 15 minutes, or until golden brown and the juices run clear when pricked. Remove the chicken from the heat and set aside.
6. In a medium pot, bring 10 oz. water to boil and add the spinach. Cook over medium heat for 10 minutes or until tender. Drain the spinach well and season with a pinch of salt and black pepper.
7. Stuff each chicken breast with the red peppers and garlic, spinach, crumbled bacon, and mozzarella cheese.
8. Lightly grease a baking sheet and place the filled chicken onto the sheet. Place in the oven and bake for 5 minutes.

INGREDIENTS

CREAMY BALSAMIC

2 tablespoons balsamic vinegar (30g)
1 tablespoon Greek yogurt (1/2 oz., 14.2g)
1/4 cup Half & Half (60.5g)
1 teaspoon lime juice (5.24g)
1/2 tablespoon grated Parmesan cheese (2.5g)

PREPARATION

CREAMY BALSAMIC:

1. Combine the balsamic vinegar, Greek yogurt, half & half, and lime juice in a medium saucepan over medium heat for 5 minutes while the chicken bakes. Frequently stir until the mixture is thoroughly combined.
2. Remove the chicken from the oven, plate, and top with the creamy balsamic sauce and the Parmesan cheese. Serve and enjoy.

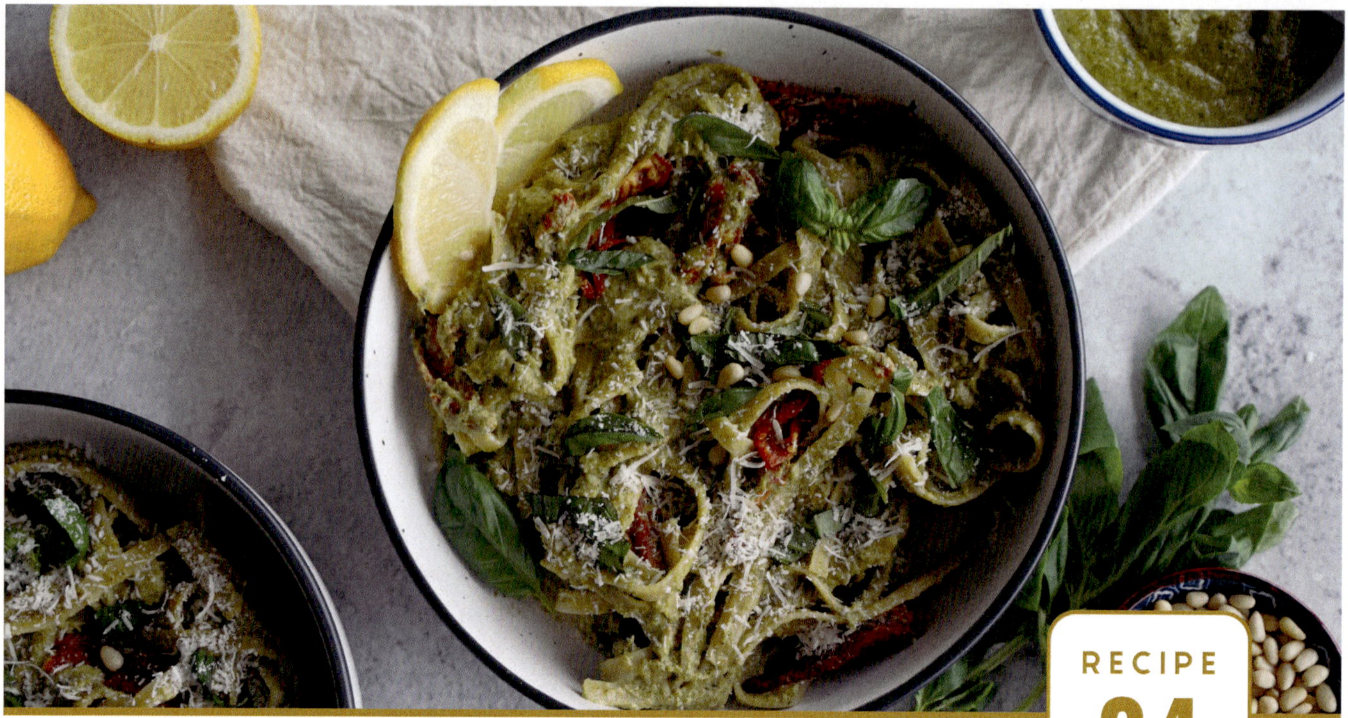

DINNER RECIPES

RECIPE 04

CREAMY PESTO PASTA

INGREDIENTS

BROCCOLI PESTO

2½ cups broccoli florets (227.5g)
2 tablespoons freshly chopped fresh basil (5.3g)
3 garlic cloves (1 tablespoon, 15g)
1/2 cup Parmesan cheese (50g)
1/4 cup pine nuts (33.8g)
1/4 teaspoon salt (1.5g)
4 tablespoons extra-virgin olive oil (56g)

PREPARATION

BROCCOLI PESTO:

1. Bring a medium pot of water to a boil. Add the broccoli and cook for 6 minutes, or until tender-crisp but still bright in color. Remove from the heat, drain, and rinse with cold water to stop the cooking.
2. Place the cooked broccoli, basil, garlic cloves, Parmesan cheese, pine nuts, and salt into a blender or food processor and pulse until finely chopped.
3. While pulsing, slowly pour in the olive oil in a thin stream.
4. Purée until smooth and transfer to a bowl. Set aside.

INGREDIENTS

CREAM SAUCE

1 tablespoon unsalted butter (14.2g)
1/2 teaspoon garlic powder (1.6g)
1/4 teaspoon salt (1.5g)
1 teaspoon black pepper (2.3g)
1 teaspoon seasoned salt (1.2g)
1/2 teaspoon Cajun seasoning (10g)
1/3 cup heavy cream (78.1g)
1/3 cup reduced-sodium chicken stock (74.8g)
1/2 cup grated Parmesan cheese (50g)
1/2 cup chopped sun-dried tomatoes (27g)
8 oz. uncooked fettuccine noodles (1/2 pound, 226.8g)
2 lemon wedges (27g)

PREPARATION

CREAM SAUCE & PASTA:

1. Bring a medium pot of water to a boil. Cook the fettuccini for about 15 minutes or until al dente. When done, drain and rinse with cold water.
2. In a medium pot over medium heat, melt the butter. Once completely melted, add the garlic powder, salt, black pepper, seasoned salt, Cajun seasoning, and whisk until smooth.
3. Slowly add the heavy cream while continually whisking. Gradually add the chicken stock and the 1/2 cup Parmesan, whisk until smooth.
4. Bring to a gentle boil, stirring constantly. Once the sauce is boiling, reduce the heat and stir in the broccoli pesto. Add the sun-dried tomatoes and simmer for 5 minutes, stirring often until the desired consistency is reached.
5. Add the cooked pasta to the sauce and stir to combine. Squeeze fresh lemon over the pasta, serve, and enjoy.

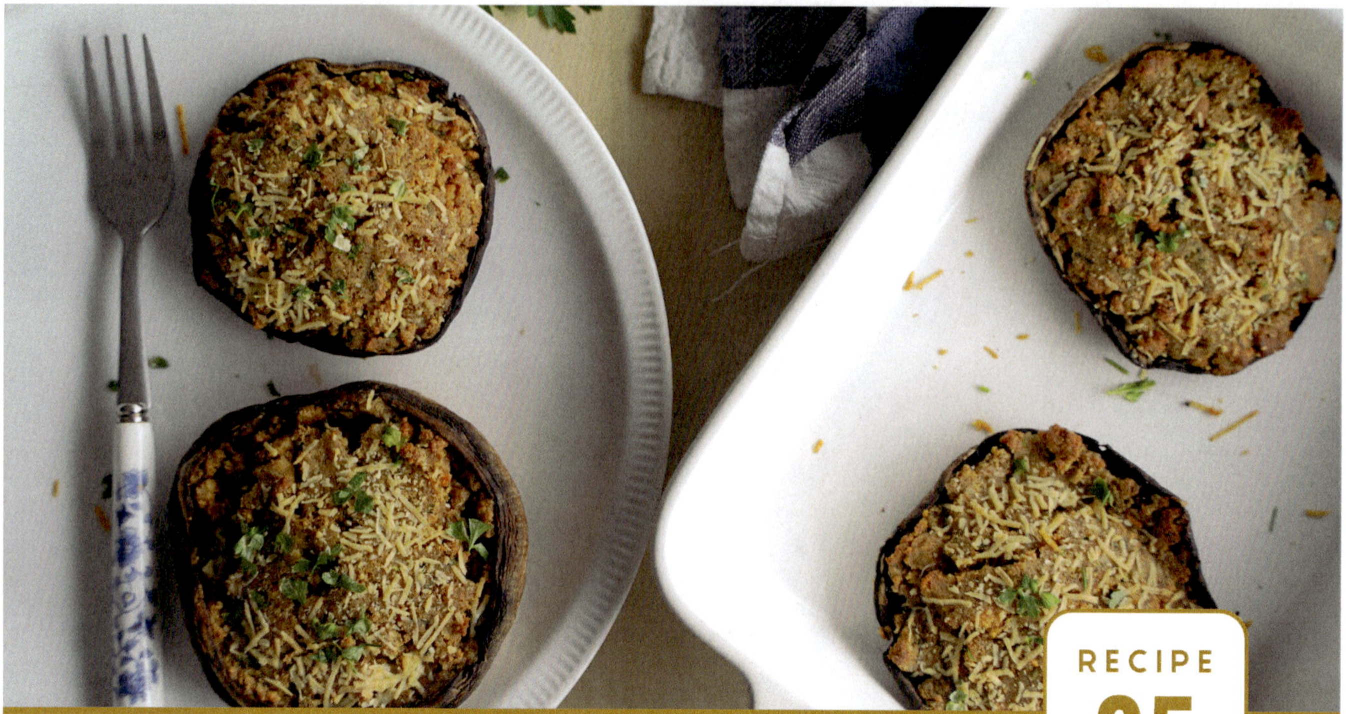

RECIPE 05

SEAFOOD-STUFFED MUSHROOMS

INGREDIENTS

2 tablespoons whole milk (30g)
1/2 a jumbo egg (31.5g)
1¼ tablespoons unsalted butter - melted (17.8g)
2.5 oz. Jiffy Corn Muffin Mix (70.9g)
1/4 tablespoon granulated sugar (3.2g)
4 fresh Portobello mushrooms (336g)
8 oz. crabmeat (226.8g)
1½ teaspoon kosher salt (9g)
1 teaspoon black pepper (2.3g)
1 teaspoon Old Bay seasoning (2.4g)
1/4 teaspoon paprika (0.6g)
1/2 teaspoon onion powder (1.2g)
4 teaspoons chopped fresh thyme (3.2g)
1½ tablespoons chopped fresh parsley (5.7g)
3 teaspoons chopped fresh chives (3g)
6 oz. cream cheese - softened, at room temperature (170.1g)
1/4 cup grated Parmesan, plus more for topping (25g)

PREPARATION

1. Preheat the oven to 375°F (190°C), and grease a 9x13-inch baking dish with butter or non-stick cooking spray.
2. In a large bowl, whisk together the milk and eggs, then whisk in the melted butter.
3. Combine the Jiffy Corn Muffin Mix and sugar. Stir the dry mixture into the egg mixture with a wooden spoon. Transfer the batter to the prepared pan.
4. Bake for 15-20 minutes, or until golden and a toothpick inserted in the center comes out clean. Cool completely, then crumble into a large bowl and set aside.
5. For the mushrooms, grease a baking sheet with cooking spray.
6. Wipe the mushrooms clean with a damp towel and remove the stems. Spoon out the gills and the base of the stem, making deep cups. Discard the gills and stems.
7. In a medium bowl, add the crabmeat, kosher salt, black pepper, Old Bay seasoning, paprika, onion powder, thyme, parsley, chives, and crumbled cornbread. Mix in the cream cheese and Parmesan cheese until well blended and creamy.
8. Fill the mushroom caps with a heaping teaspoon of filling, and place on the baking sheet. Sprinkle the tops with Parmesan and bake for 15 - 20 minutes, or until the mushrooms are soft and the tops are golden brown. Allow to cool for 5 minutes before serving.

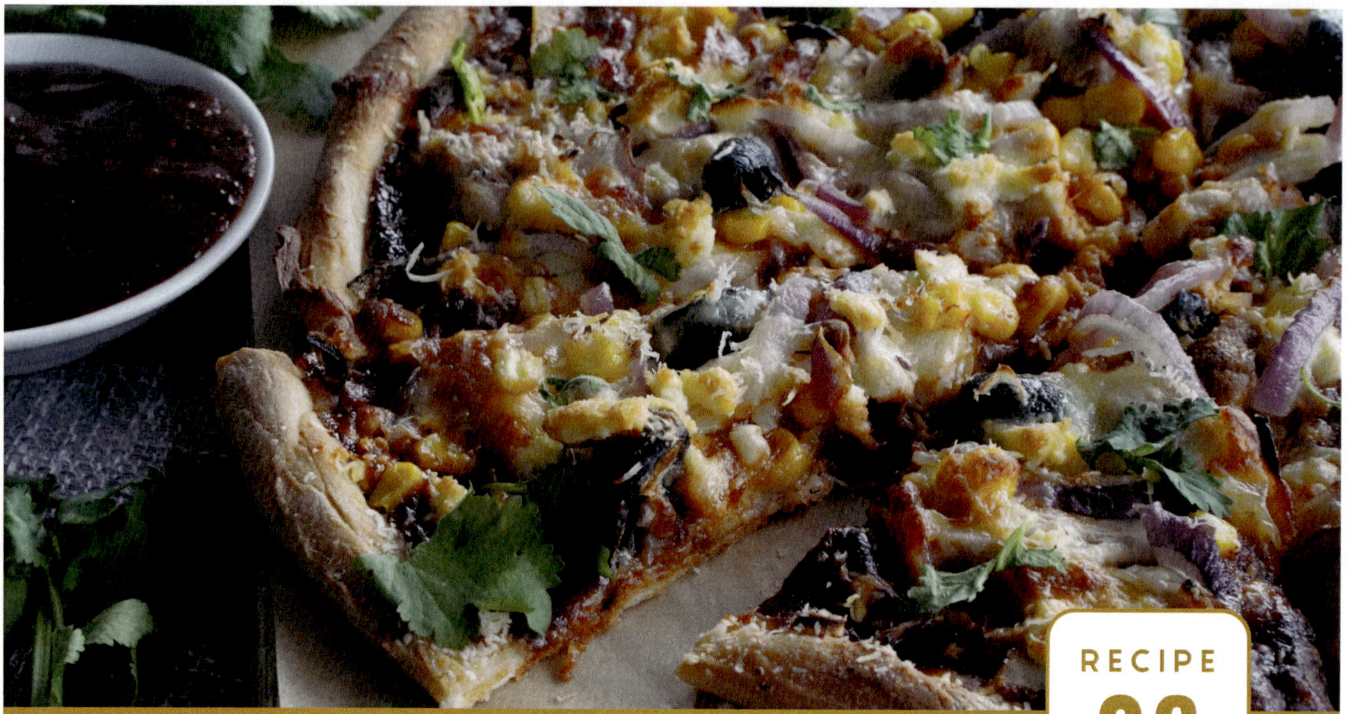

RECIPE 06

BARBEQUE CHICKEN PIZZA

INGREDIENTS

DOUGH

1 can Pillsbury Classic Pizza Crust (13.8 oz., 391.2g)

1 tablespoon extra-virgin olive oil (14g)

PREPARATION

DOUGH:

1. Preheat the oven to 425°F (220°C).
2. Sprinkle cornmeal on a cutting board or another work surface. Unroll the dough onto the cornmeal. Starting at the center, press the dough into a 12-inch circle and form a 1/2-inch rim. Spray or grease a 15x10-inch or larger dark or non-stick cookie sheet, and carefully transfer the pizza dough to the pan.
3. To prevent the pizza toppings from making your pizza crust soggy, brush the shaped dough lightly with the extra virgin olive oil. Using your fingers or a fork, push dents into the surface of the dough to prevent bubbling.

INGREDIENTS

BARBEQUE SAUCE AND PIZZA

1 cup Sweet Baby Ray's barbeque sauce (280g)
1/2 cup Open Pit barbeque sauce (137g)
1/4 cup orange juice (62g)
1/2 tablespoon lemon juice (7.1g)
1 teaspoon unsalted butter (4.8g)
1½ teaspoons onion powder (3g)
1/2 teaspoon garlic powder (1.6g)
Pinch of salt
1 tablespoon apple butter(16g), [or combine 1½ tablespoons natural apple sauce (21.3g), 1/2 tablespoon dark brown sugar - packed (6g),1 teaspoon cinnamon (2.6g) and 1 teaspoon honey (6.9g)]
1 cup shredded mozzarella cheese (112g)
1/3 cup crumbled feta cheese (49.5g)
1/2 cup sliced red onion (74g)
1/4 cup drained black olives (64g)
1/2 cup drained canned corn (82g)
1 cup cooked and shredded chicken (8 oz., 226.8g)
1/4 cup grated parmesan cheese (25g)
1 tablespoon chopped fresh cilantro (7.1g)

PREPARATION

BARBEQUE SAUCE AND PIZZA:

1. In a medium pot over medium-low heat, mix the Sweet Baby Ray's barbeque sauce, Open Pit barbeque sauce, orange juice, lemon juice, butter, onion powder, garlic powder, salt, and apple butter (or apple sauce mixture). Simmer for 10 minutes until completely smooth and combined.
2. Spread the desired amount of barbeque sauce mixture over the crust to within 1/2 inch of the edge. Top with the mozzarella cheese, feta cheese, red onions, olives, corn, and shredded chicken. Sprinkle with Parmesan cheese.
3. Bake the pizza for 14-18 minutes, or until the crust is golden brown and the cheese is melted.
4. Remove from the oven and top with fresh cilantro (if desired). Slice hot pizza and serve.

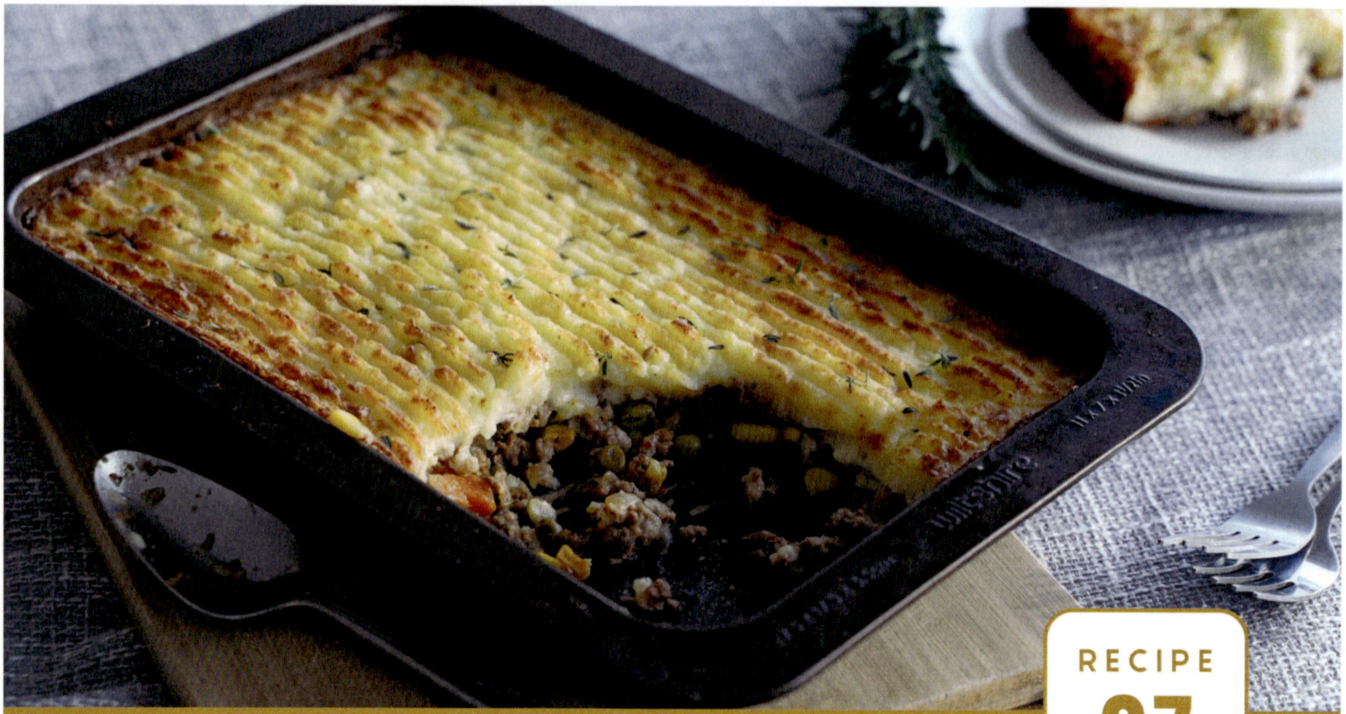

RECIPE
07

SHEPHERD'S PIE (TURKEY)

INGREDIENTS

3 tablespoons unsalted butter (42.6g)
1/2 cup chopped onions (80g)
1/4 cup diced carrots (32g)
12 oz. 85/15% ground turkey (3/4 pound, 340.2g)
1/4 teaspoon lemon pepper (0.7g)
1/4 teaspoon garlic powder (0.8g)
1/4 teaspoon salt (1.5g)
1/4 teaspoon black pepper (0.6g)
Light sprinkle of crushed red pepper flakes
1/4 teaspoon dried parsley (0.1g)
1/4 teaspoon dried thyme (0.3g)
1/4 teaspoon dried rosemary (0.3g)
1/2 teaspoon Worcestershire sauce (2.9g)
1/4 cup beef broth (60g)
1/4 cup peas (33.5g)
1/4 cup corn (41g)
1 pound peeled and quartered white potatoes (about 2 large potatoes, (453.6g)
1/2 cup Half & Half (121g)
1/2 cup shredded cheddar cheese (56.5g)

PREPARATION

1. In a large skillet over medium heat, melt 1 tablespoon of the butter. Once melted, add the onions and carrots, and sauté for 6-10 minutes, or until tender.
2. Add the ground turkey, lemon pepper, garlic powder, salt, black pepper, crushed red pepper, dried parsley, dried thyme, and dried rosemary; cook for 15 minutes or until the meat is browned and juices run clear.
3. Add the Worcestershire sauce, beef broth, peas, and corn, and simmer for 5-10 minutes.
4. While the meat is cooking, prepare a large pot of water for the potatoes. Add a pinch of salt to the water, and bring to a boil over medium-high heat.
5. Preheat the oven to 400°F (205°C).
6. Add the potatoes to the water, bring the water back to a boil, then reduce the heat to medium and cook for 20 minutes or until the potatoes are tender. Drain the water, leaving the potatoes in the pot.
7. Add the half & half, cheddar cheese, and 2 tablespoons of butter to the potatoes and mash with a fork/potato masher.
8. Spread the meat mixture evenly over the bottom of a 9x13-inch baking dish. Carefully spread the mashed potatoes over the top of the meat, making sure to cover it completely.
9. Rough the mashed potatoes surface with a fork, forming peaks to allow optimal browning.
10. Bake for 30 minutes, or until browned and bubbling. If necessary, set the oven to broil for the last few minutes to help the surface of the mashed potatoes brown.
11. Allow to cool for 10 minutes before serving.

NICK'S NUTRITIONAL NUGGETS

The "Shepherd's Pie" in this cookbook is Cottage Pie. As shepherd's pie is an Irish specialty dish made with ground lamb, whereas cottage pie is an English dish made with ground beef or any ground meat. The terms have become interchangeable throughout the 20th century, despite the difference in origin and ingredients.

nutrition facts dinner

Rosemary Gravy Chicken Pot Pie

Nutrition Facts

4 servings per container
Serving size **1 pie (0.0g)**

Amount Per Serving	
Calories	**480**
	% Daily Value*
Total Fat 28g	**36%**
Saturated Fat 13g	**65%**
Trans Fat 2g	
Cholesterol 55mg	**18%**
Sodium 510mg	**22%**
Total Carbohydrate 45g	**16%**
Dietary Fiber 3g	**11%**
Total Sugars 6g	
Includes 0g Added Sugars	**0%**
Protein 14g	
Vitamin D 0mcg	0%
Calcium 50mg	4%
Iron 1.7mg	10%
Potassium 280mg	6%

* The % Daily Value (DV) tells you how much a nutrient in a serving of food contributes to a daily diet. 2,000 calories a day is used for general nutrition advice.

Pink Enchiladas

Nutrition Facts

4 servings per container
Serving size **2.35oz (0.0g)**

Amount Per Serving	
Calories	**610**
	% Daily Value*
Total Fat 44g	**56%**
Saturated Fat 16g	**80%**
Trans Fat 1g	
Cholesterol 105mg	**35%**
Sodium 1520mg	**66%**
Total Carbohydrate 29g	**11%**
Dietary Fiber 5g	**18%**
Total Sugars 6g	
Includes 0g Added Sugars	**0%**
Protein 25g	
Vitamin D 0.3mcg	2%
Calcium 390mg	30%
Iron 2.2mg	10%
Potassium 350mg	8%

* The % Daily Value (DV) tells you how much a nutrient in a serving of food contributes to a daily diet. 2,000 calories a day is used for general nutrition advice.

Balsamic Stuffed Chicken Taco

Nutrition Facts

6 servings per container
Serving size **1 slice (0.0g)**

Amount Per Serving	
Calories	**500**
	% Daily Value*
Total Fat 17g	**22%**
Saturated Fat 7g	**35%**
Trans Fat 0g	
Cholesterol 60mg	**20%**
Sodium 1510mg	**66%**
Total Carbohydrate 67g	**24%**
Dietary Fiber 2g	**7%**
Total Sugars 30g	
Includes 17g Added Sugars	**34%**
Protein 21g	
Vitamin D 0.1mcg	0%
Calcium 190mg	15%
Iron 2.5mg	15%
Potassium 340mg	8%

* The % Daily Value (DV) tells you how much a nutrient in a serving of food contributes to a daily diet. 2,000 calories a day is used for general nutrition advice.

Creamy Pesto Pasta

Nutrition Facts

4 servings per container
Serving size **2 oz (0.0g)**

Amount Per Serving	
Calories	**580**
	% Daily Value*
Total Fat 45g	**58%**
Saturated Fat 16g	**80%**
Trans Fat 0.5g	
Cholesterol 80mg	**27%**
Sodium 3010mg	**131%**
Total Carbohydrate 31g	**11%**
Dietary Fiber 4g	**14%**
Total Sugars 10g	
Includes 0g Added Sugars	**0%**
Protein 18g	
Vitamin D 0.4mcg	2%
Calcium 300mg	25%
Iron 3.7mg	20%
Potassium 580mg	10%

* The % Daily Value (DV) tells you how much a nutrient in a serving of food contributes to a daily diet. 2,000 calories a day is used for general nutrition advice.

nutrition facts dinner

Seafood-Stuffed Mushrooms

Nutrition Facts

4 servings per container
Serving size 1 Mushrooms (0.0g)

Amount Per Serving	
Calories	**470**
	% Daily Value*
Total Fat 35g	**45%**
Saturated Fat 15g	**75%**
Trans Fat 1g	
Cholesterol 145mg	**48%**
Sodium 1590mg	**69%**
Total Carbohydrate 21g	**8%**
Dietary Fiber 2g	**7%**
Total Sugars 8g	
Includes 4g Added Sugars	**8%**
Protein 20g	
Vitamin D 0.4mcg	2%
Calcium 210mg	15%
Iron 1.8mg	10%
Potassium 610mg	15%

* The % Daily Value (DV) tells you how much a nutrient in a serving of food contributes to a daily diet. 2,000 calories a day is used for general nutrition advice.

Barbeque Chicken Pizza

Nutrition Facts

6 servings per container
Serving size 1 slice (0.0g)

Amount Per Serving	
Calories	**510**
	% Daily Value*
Total Fat 17g	**22%**
Saturated Fat 7g	**35%**
Trans Fat 0g	
Cholesterol 60mg	**20%**
Sodium 1510mg	**66%**
Total Carbohydrate 69g	**25%**
Dietary Fiber 3g	**11%**
Total Sugars 32g	
Includes 19g Added Sugars	**38%**
Protein 21g	
Vitamin D 0.1mcg	0%
Calcium 190mg	15%
Iron 2.6mg	15%
Potassium 340mg	8%

* The % Daily Value (DV) tells you how much a nutrient in a serving of food contributes to a daily diet. 2,000 calories a day is used for general nutrition advice.

Shepherd's Pie (Turkey)

Nutrition Facts

About 3 servings per container
Serving size 2 cups (0.0g)

Amount Per Serving	
Calories	**600**
	% Daily Value*
Total Fat 37g	**47%**
Saturated Fat 18g	**90%**
Trans Fat 1g	
Cholesterol 150mg	**50%**
Sodium 570mg	**25%**
Total Carbohydrate 40g	**15%**
Dietary Fiber 4g	**14%**
Total Sugars 6g	
Includes 0g Added Sugars	**0%**
Protein 29g	
Vitamin D 0.5mcg	2%
Calcium 250mg	20%
Iron 2.6mg	15%
Potassium 930mg	20%

* The % Daily Value (DV) tells you how much a nutrient in a serving of food contributes to a daily diet. 2,000 calories a day is used for general nutrition advice.

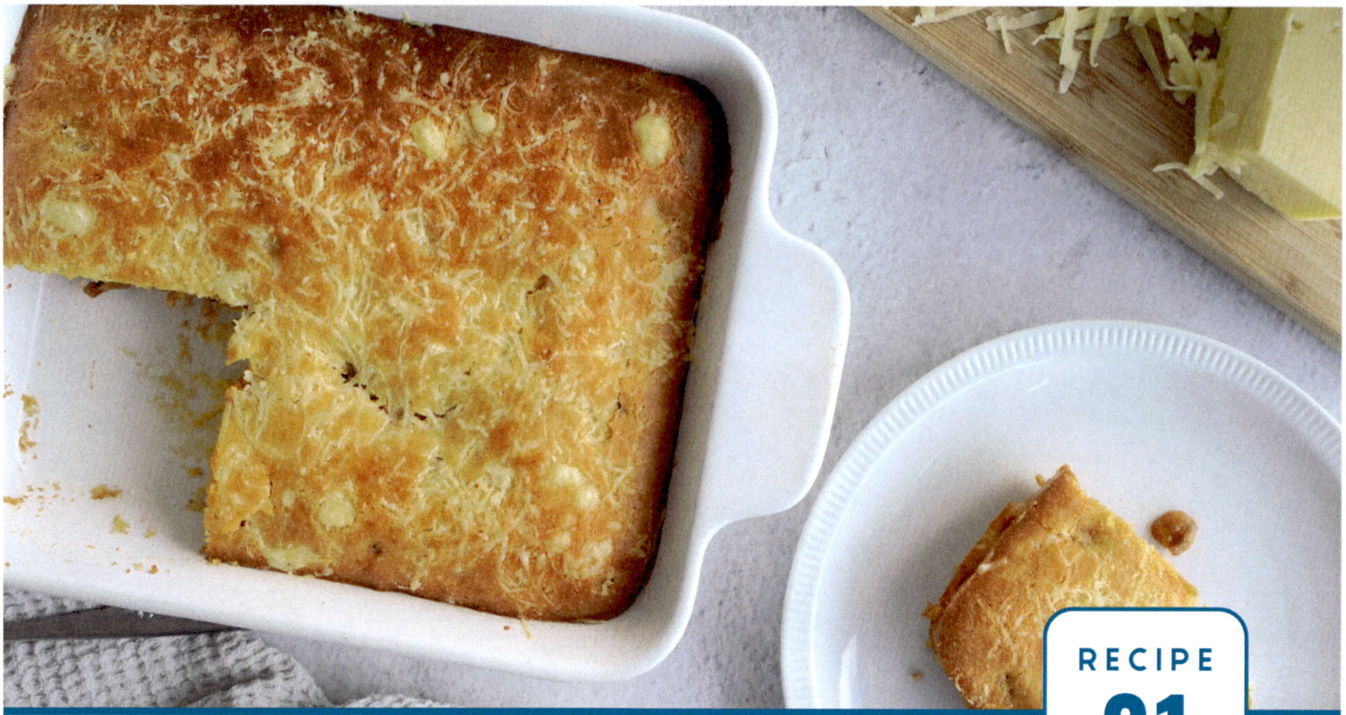

RECIPE 01

BOLD CORNBREAD

INGREDIENTS

1 pound 80/20% ground beef (453.6g)
3 tablespoons taco seasoning (25.7g)
1 package Jiffy Corn Muffin Mix (8.5 oz., 241g)
1/4 cup whole milk (61g)
2 large eggs (100g)
1 can cream-style corn (14.8 oz., 482g)
1/2 cup chunky salsa - any brand (4 oz., 113.4g)
1/4 cup shredded cheddar cheese (28g)

PREPARATION

1. Preheat the oven to 350°F (175°C).
2. In a large skillet over medium-high heat, brown the ground beef with the taco seasoning, stirring constantly.
3. In a medium bowl, combine the corn muffin mix, milk, and eggs. Mix until the batter is a smooth consistency with no lumps.
4. Spray a 9x9-inch baking pan with non-stick cooking oil spray and spread half of the cornbread batter in the bottom of the pan.
5. Combine the ground beef, corn, and salsa in a new medium bowl. Then spread on top of the cornbread batter in the pan.
6. Using a spatula, spread the remaining cornbread batter over the meat mixture, ensuring the layers are smooth.
7. Sprinkle the cheese on top of the cornbread batter.
8. Bake for 30-35 minutes, or until the top of the cornbread is golden brown. Cool for 15 minutes before serving.

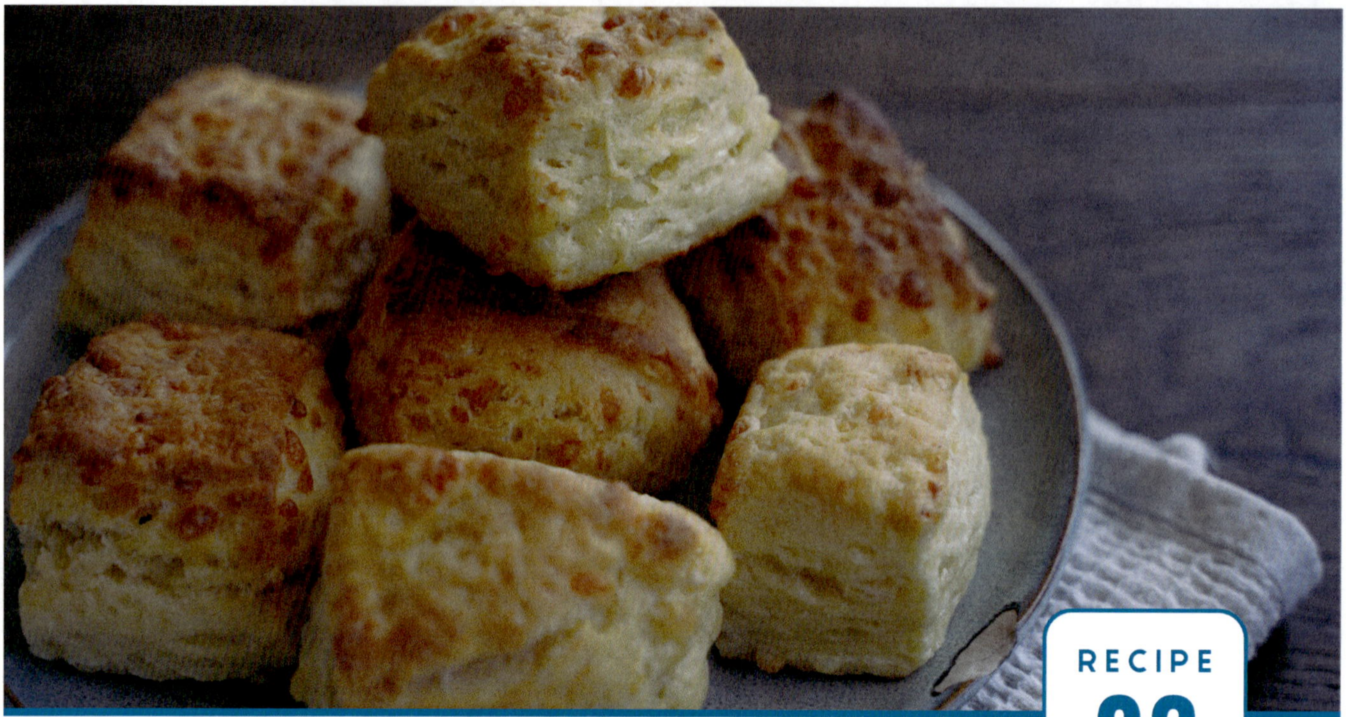

RECIPE
02

SAGE BUTTER CHEDDAR BISCUITS

INGREDIENTS

2 cups all-purpose flour - plus more for dusting (250g)
6 teaspoons baking powder - non-aluminum (30g)
1 tablespoon granulated sugar (12.6g)
1 teaspoon salt (6g)
5 tablespoons frozen unsalted butter - preferably European-style (71g)
1 cup whole milk (244g)
1/2 cup shredded Colby & Monterrey Jack cheese (4 oz., 112g)
1 garlic clove - crushed and chopped (1 teaspoon, 5g)
1/4 cup coarsely chopped sage leaves (8g)
1/8 teaspoon ground black pepper (0.3g)

PREPARATION

1. Sift the flour, baking powder, sugar, and salt into a large mixing bowl.
2. Grate 3 tablespoons of the butter and refreeze for 15 minutes.
3. Gently add the butter, milk, and shredded cheese to the flour mixture, and stir with a fork until it forms a rough ball.
4. On a well-floured surface, turn the dough out and pat it down into a rough rectangle, about an inch thick.
5. Fold the dough over and gently pat it down again. Repeat 3 times. Cover the dough loosely with a kitchen towel and allow it to rest for 30 minutes. While the dough is resting, pre-heat the oven to 425°F (220°C).
6. Gently pat out the rested dough to a rectangle that is roughly 6x10-inches in size.
7. Cut the dough into 1.5x1.5-inch square biscuits using a serrated knife. Make sure to pull the knife gently through the dough, not smashing the edges of the biscuits. (This creates dense biscuits).
8. Place the biscuits on a cookie sheet spaced at least an inch apart and bake for 15 minutes, or until golden brown. Remove from the oven and leave to cool slightly.
9. While the biscuits bake, make the sage butter. In a medium saucepan over medium-low heat, melt the remaining 2 tablespoons of butter.
10. When the butter begins to bubble slightly, add the chopped garlic clove and cook for 1 minute.
11. Add the chopped sage to the garlic butter and continue to cook, stirring, for 1-2 additional minutes, just until the butter has turned very light brown and has a rich, nutty aroma. Remove from the heat, season with ground black pepper and leave to cool slightly.
12. Once the biscuits are baked and slightly cooled, coat them with the sage butter using a pastry brush. Serve immediately and enjoy.

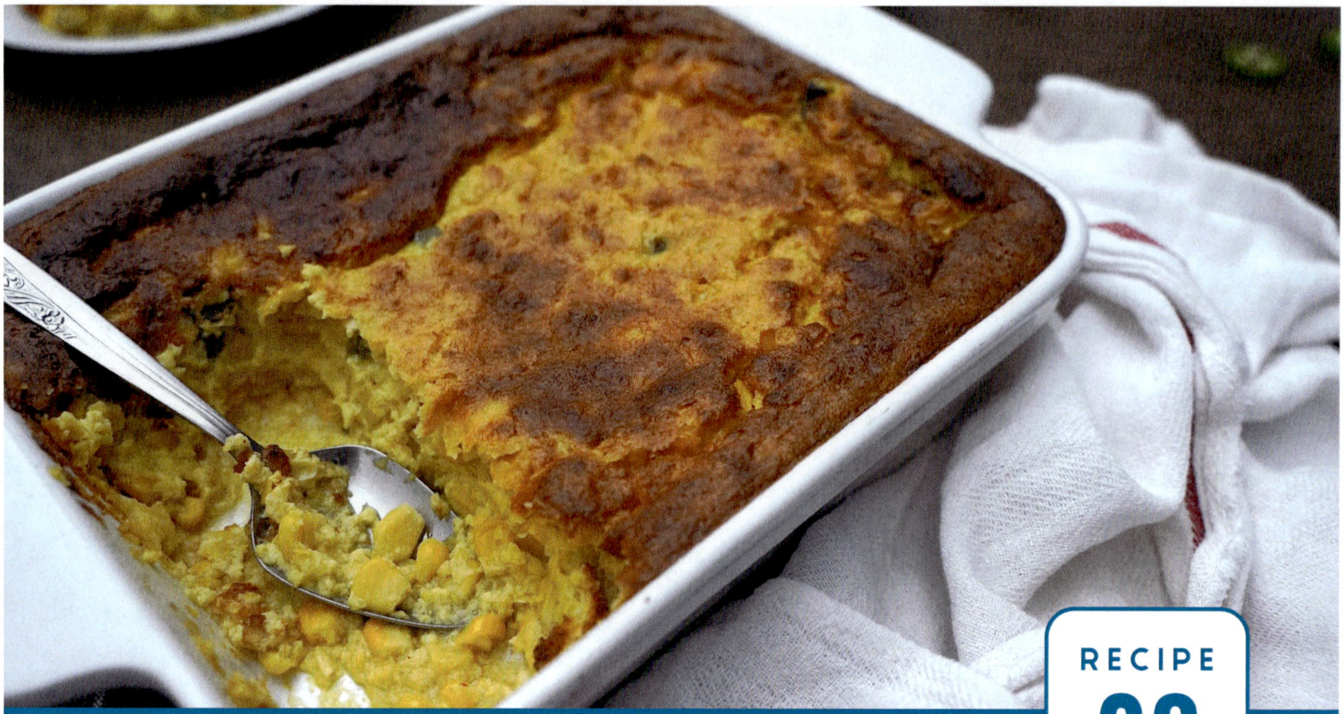

RECIPE 03

JALAPENO POPPER CORN SOUFFLÉ

INGREDIENTS

4 jumbo eggs (252g), at room temperature
2-12 oz. cans whole kernel corn - drained (422g)
2-12 oz. cans cream-style corn (964g)
1 tablespoon granulated sugar (12.6g)
1/4 cup all-purpose flour (31.3g)
1/4 cup whole milk (61g)
1/2 cup shredded mild cheddar cheese (56g)
1/2 cup chopped jalapenos (45g)
1/2 cup cream cheese (4 oz., 113.4g), at room temperature

PREPARATION

1. Preheat the oven to 350°F (175°C).
2. Separate the eggs into yolks and whites.
3. Combine the corn, creamed corn, sugar, flour, milk, cheese, chopped jalapenos, cream cheese, and egg yolks (*not egg whites*) and mix well.
4. In another bowl, whip the egg whites to soft peaks. Gently fold them into the mixture from step 3 with a rubber spatula.
5. Pour the mixture into a greased 2-quart baking dish.
6. Bake for 1-1½ hours or until a toothpick inserted in the center comes out clean. Let it cool for 15 minutes before serving.

NOTES:

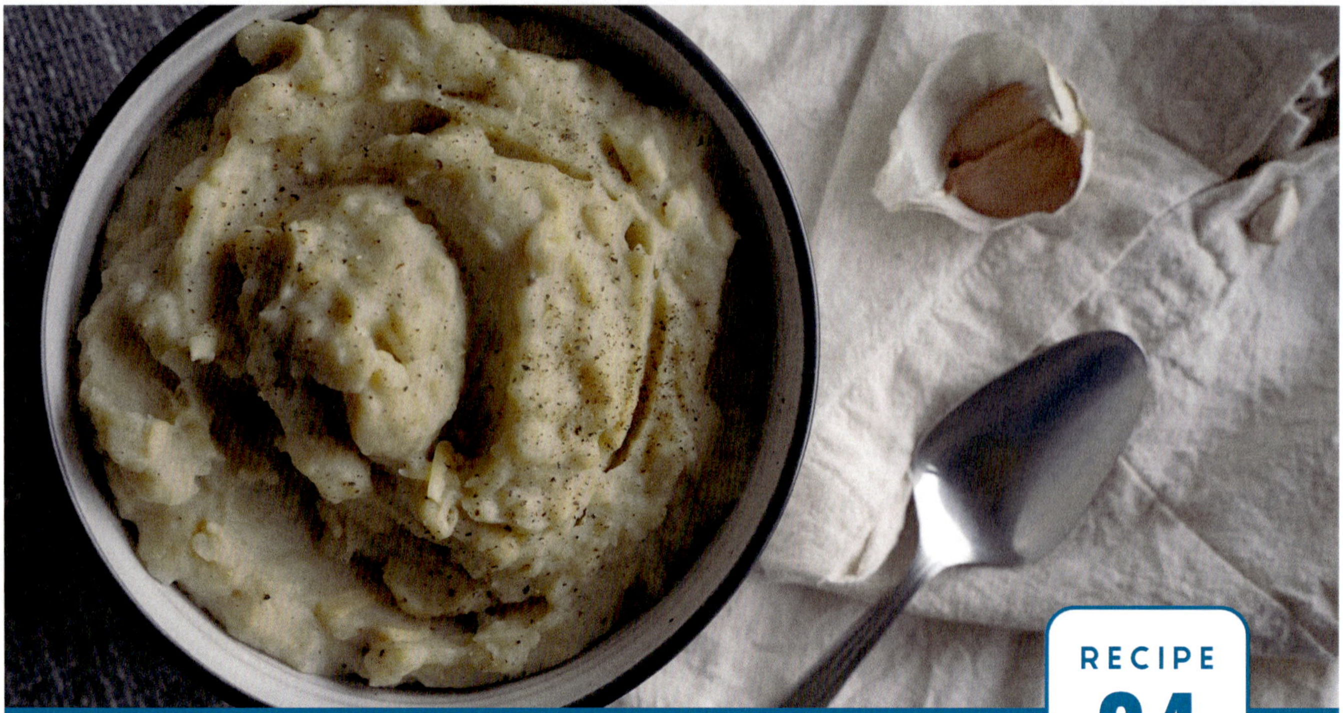

RECIPE 04

SMOKED GOUDA GARLIC MASHED POTATOES

INGREDIENTS

3 garlic cloves - unpeeled (1 tablespoon, 15g)
1 tablespoon extra-virgin olive oil (14g)
2 pounds peeled and quartered Russet potatoes (about 6 potatoes, 907.2g)
1/2 cup shredded smoked Gouda (4 oz., 113.4g)
4 tablespoons unsalted butter - softened (56.8g)
1/2 cup whole milk (122g)
1 teaspoon salt (6g)
1 teaspoon black pepper (2.3g)

PREPARATION

1. Preheat the oven to 350°F (175°C).
2. Place the garlic cloves on a piece of aluminum foil and drizzle with olive oil.
3. Bake the garlic for 15-20 minutes or until the cloves, are tender and browned.
4. In a large pot, add water and a dash of salt and bring to a boil.
5. Add the potatoes and cook for about 30 minutes, or until fork-tender.
6. Drain the potatoes, transfer them to a large bowl and mash them.
7. Add the smoked Gouda, butter, milk, salt, and black pepper to the potatoes, and mix thoroughly.
8. Remove the garlic from the oven, and cut it in half.
9. Crumble the softened cloves into the potato mixture.
10. Blend the potatoes with an electric hand mixer until creamy or until the desired consistency is achieved. Add milk to adjust consistency, if needed. Serve immediately.

NOTES:

nutrition facts dinner sides

Bold Cornbread

Nutrition Facts

6 servings per container
Serving size 1 slice (0.0g)

Amount Per Serving	
Calories	**490**
	% Daily Value*
Total Fat 24g	**31%**
Saturated Fat 9g	**45%**
Trans Fat 1g	
Cholesterol 125mg	**42%**
Sodium 1120mg	**49%**
Total Carbohydrate 48g	**17%**
Dietary Fiber 3g	**11%**
Total Sugars 12g	
Includes 7g Added Sugars	**14%**
Protein 20g	
Vitamin D 0.4mcg	2%
Calcium 130mg	10%
Iron 3.5mg	20%
Potassium 390mg	8%

* The % Daily Value (DV) tells you how much a nutrient in a serving of food contributes to a daily diet. 2,000 calories a day is used for general nutrition advice.

Sage Butter Cheddar Biscuits

Nutrition Facts

8 servings per container
Serving size 1 biscuit (0.0g)

Amount Per Serving	
Calories	**260**
	% Daily Value*
Total Fat 13g	**17%**
Saturated Fat 8g	**40%**
Trans Fat 0g	
Cholesterol 35mg	**12%**
Sodium 400mg	**17%**
Total Carbohydrate 30g	**11%**
Dietary Fiber 1g	**4%**
Total Sugars 3g	
Includes 2g Added Sugars	**4%**
Protein 8g	
Vitamin D 0mcg	0%
Calcium 350mg	25%
Iron 2.1mg	10%
Potassium 490mg	10%

* The % Daily Value (DV) tells you how much a nutrient in a serving of food contributes to a daily diet. 2,000 calories a day is used for general nutrition advice.

Jalapeno Popper Corn Soufflé

Nutrition Facts

6 servings per container
Serving size 1 4x4 square (0.0g)

Amount Per Serving	
Calories	**360**
	% Daily Value*
Total Fat 15g	**19%**
Saturated Fat 7g	**35%**
Trans Fat 0g	
Polyunsaturated Fat 2g	
Monounsaturated Fat 4.5g	
Cholesterol 185mg	**62%**
Sodium 750mg	**33%**
Total Carbohydrate 48g	**17%**
Dietary Fiber 4g	**14%**
Total Sugars 12g	
Includes 2g Added Sugars	**4%**
Protein 14g	
Vitamin D 0.9mcg	4%
Calcium 130mg	10%
Iron 1.8mg	10%
Potassium 430mg	10%

* The % Daily Value (DV) tells you how much a nutrient in a serving of food contributes to a daily diet. 2,000 calories a day is used for general nutrition advice.

Smoked Gouda Garlic Mashed Potatoes

Nutrition Facts

4 servings per container
Serving size 1/2 cup (0.0g)

Amount Per Serving	
Calories	**450**
	% Daily Value*
Total Fat 24g	**31%**
Saturated Fat 13g	**65%**
Trans Fat 0g	
Cholesterol 50mg	**17%**
Sodium 990mg	**43%**
Total Carbohydrate 48g	**17%**
Dietary Fiber 5g	**18%**
Total Sugars 4g	
Includes 0g Added Sugars	**0%**
Protein 11g	
Vitamin D 0mcg	0%
Calcium 260mg	20%
Iron 0.8mg	4%
Potassium 800mg	15%

* The % Daily Value (DV) tells you how much a nutrient in a serving of food contributes to a daily diet. 2,000 calories a day is used for general nutrition advice.

Figs aren't fruits,
they are flowers.

DID YOU KNOW?

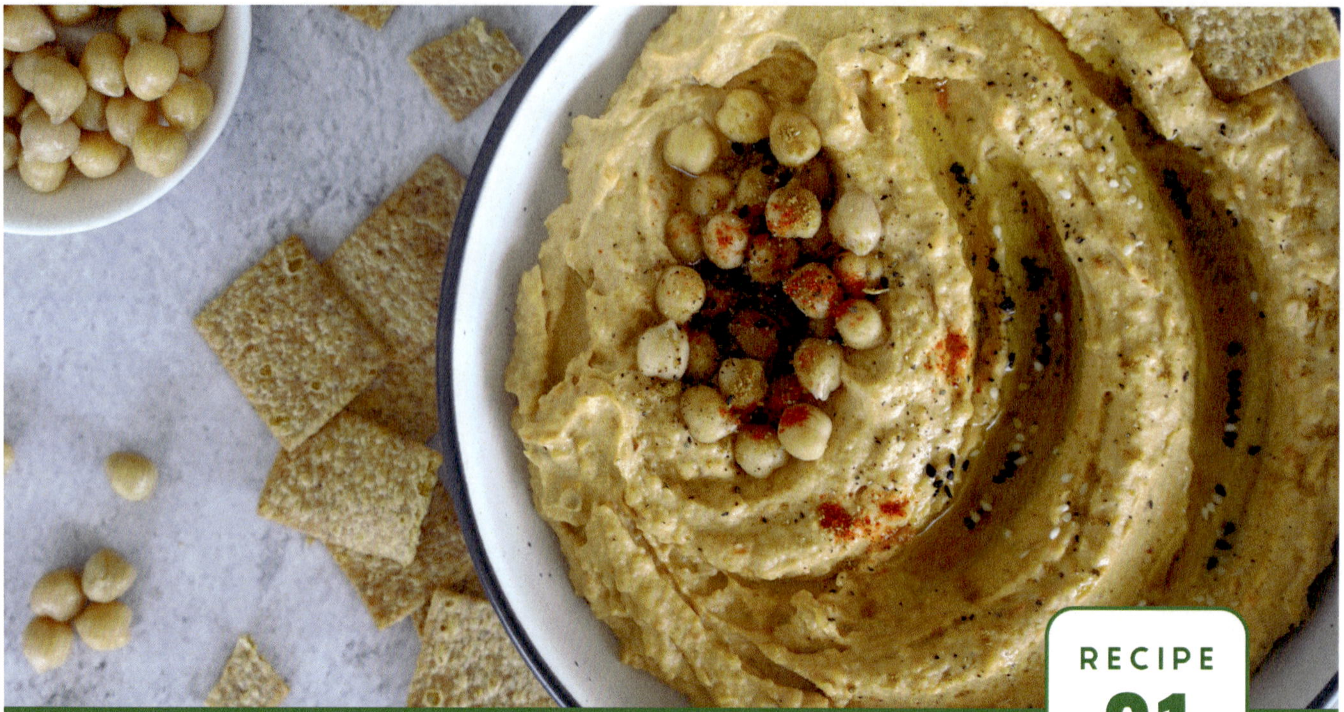

RECIPE 01

SNACKS RECIPES

SWEET POTATO HUMMUS

INGREDIENTS

2 cups chopped sweet potatoes (266g)
1/4 cup extra-virgin olive oil (54g)
1/2 teaspoon kosher salt (3g)
1/2 teaspoon black pepper (1.2g)
8 oz. canned chickpeas - drained, reserve liquid (226.8g)
1/2 cup tahini (120g)
1/4 cup lemon juice (61g)
1 tablespoon cumin (6g)

PREPARATION

1. Preheat the oven to 450°F (220°C).
2. On a large baking sheet, toss the sweet potatoes with the olive oil, kosher salt, and black pepper.
3. Roast the potatoes for about 20 minutes or until tender. Toss halfway through. When tender, remove from the oven and leave to cool.
4. Put the sweet potatoes, chickpeas, tahini, lemon juice, and cumin into a large bowl and toss to combine. Transfer the mixture to a food processor and blend until smooth. Use the reserved chickpea liquid to thin the consistency, if needed.
5. Taste and adjust (sparingly) the salt and black pepper to taste. Serve and enjoy.

NOTES:

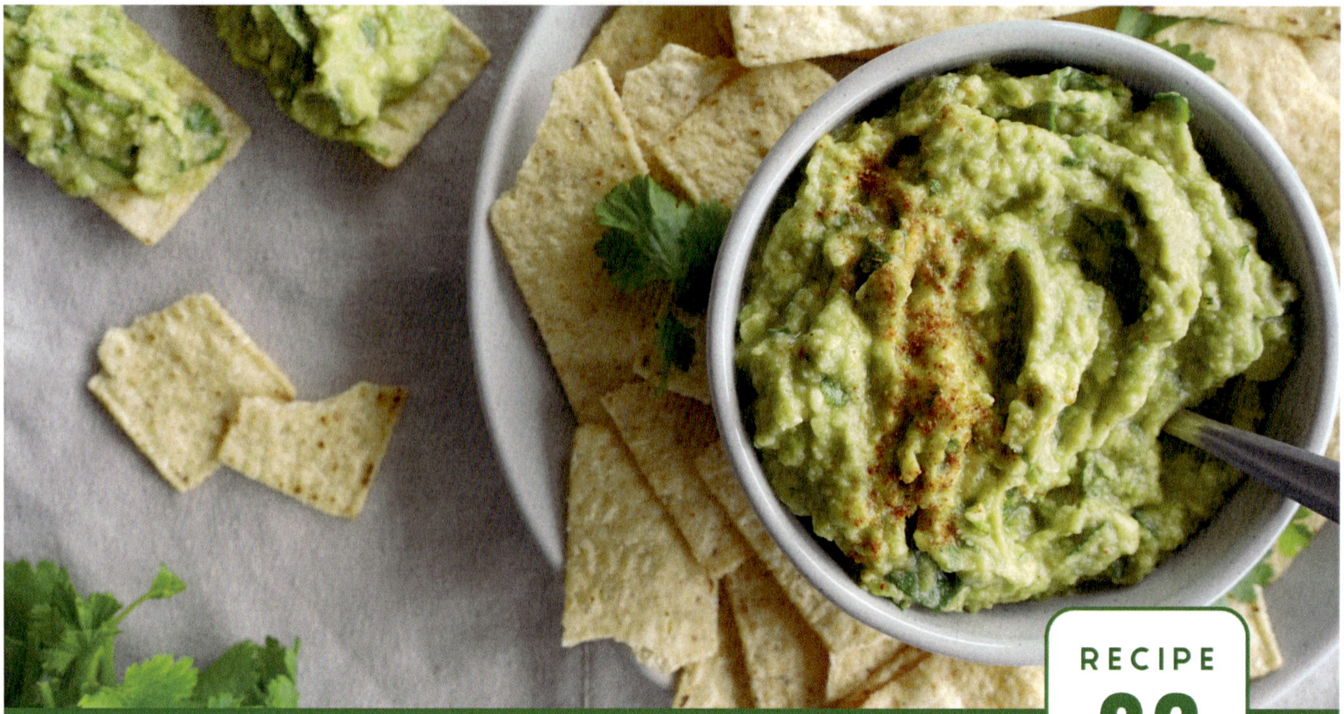

RECIPE 02

SWEET & SPICY GUACAMOLE

SNACKS RECIPES

INGREDIENTS

4 cups avocado - pitted and mashed (920g)
1/2 cup lime juice (121g)
1/2 teaspoon kosher salt (3g)
1/2 teaspoon black pepper (1.2g)
1/2 teaspoon ground cinnamon (1.3g)
1/2 tablespoon onion powder (3.5g)
1/2 teaspoon garlic powder (1.6g)
1/4 teaspoon Cajun seasoning (5g)
3 tablespoons chopped fresh cilantro (42.5g)
1½ tablespoons honey (31.5g)
Pinch ground cayenne pepper

PREPARATION

1. Put the mashed avocados, lime juice, salt, black pepper, cinnamon, onion powder, garlic powder, and Cajun seasoning in a medium bowl and use a fork to combine.
2. Add the cilantro, honey, and cayenne pepper to the avocado mixture and mix well.
3. Place a layer of plastic wrap on the top of the guacamole bowl, to prevent browning. Refrigerate for 1 hour for the best flavor, or serve immediately and enjoy.

NOTES:

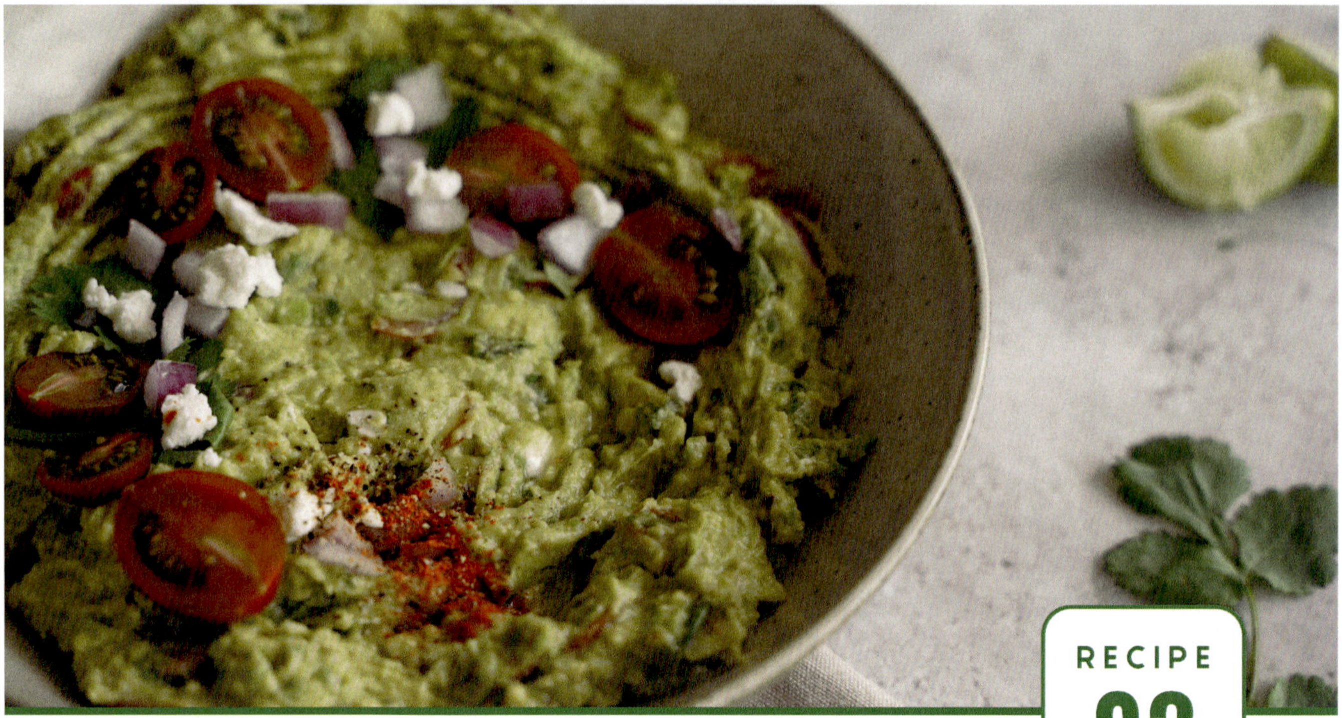

RECIPE 03

GOAT CHEESE GUACAMOLE

INGREDIENTS

4 cups avocado - pitted and mashed (920g)
1/2 cup lime juice (121g)
1/2 teaspoon kosher salt (3g)
1/2 teaspoon black pepper (1.2g)
1 oz. goat cheese – crumbled (28.4g)
3 tablespoons chopped fresh cilantro (42.5g)
1/2 cup diced red onion (74g)
2 cups diced roma (plum) tomatoes (298g)
1 teaspoon minced garlic (5g)
Pinch ground cayenne pepper (optional)*

PREPARATION

1. Put the mashed avocado, lime juice, salt, black pepper, and goat cheese in a medium bowl and mix well with a fork.
2. Add the cilantro, onion, tomatoes, and garlic to the avocado mixture and mix well. If using, add the cayenne pepper here as well.
3. Place a layer of plastic wrap on the top of the bowl with the guacamole to prevent browning. Refrigerate for 1 hour for the best flavor, or serve immediately and enjoy.

NOTES:

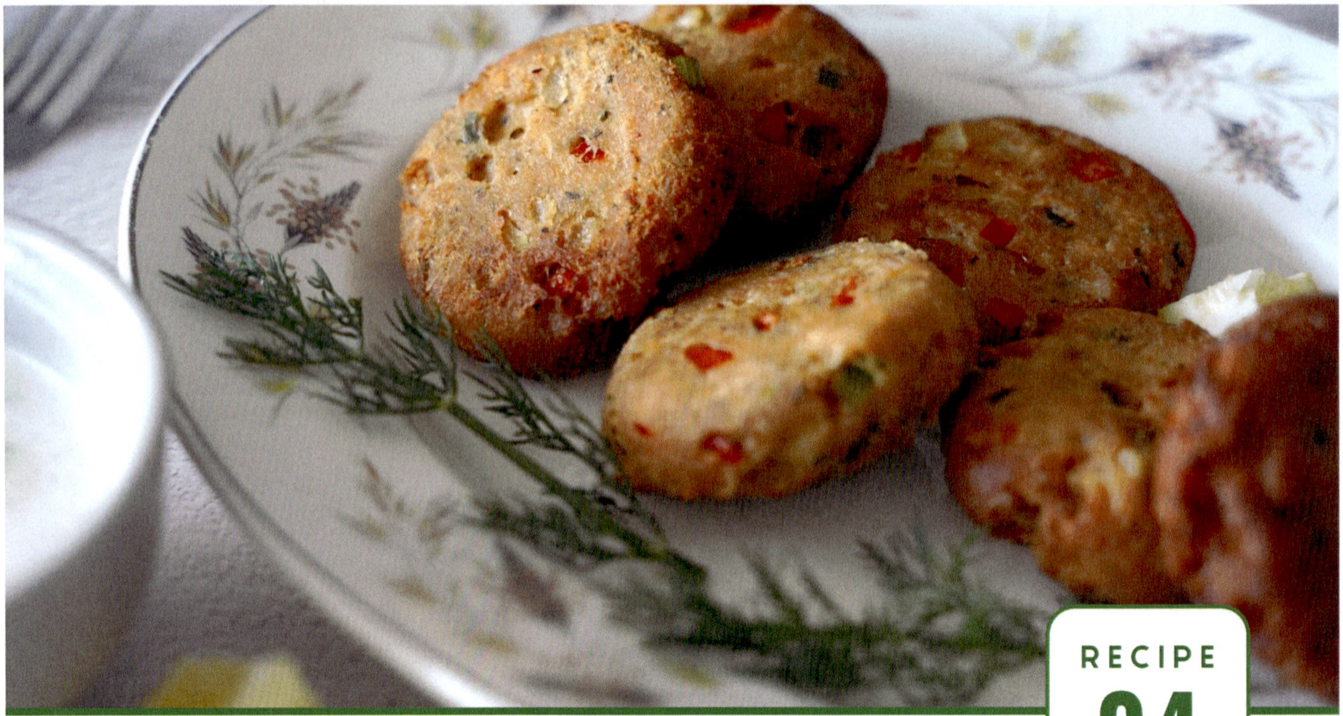

RECIPE 04

CAJUN SALMON CROQUETTES

SNACKS RECIPES

INGREDIENTS

15 oz. can wild salmon - drained (425g)
2 jumbo eggs - beaten (126g)
2 tablespoons diced green onion (12g)
1/2 cup diced sweet yellow onion (82.8g)
1/2 cup diced bell pepper (74.5g)
1 tablespoon Cajun seasoning (60g)
1/2 cup bread crumbs (54g)
Vegetable Oil - for frying
A squeeze of fresh lemon

PREPARATION

1. Put the salmon, eggs, green and yellow onions, bell peppers, Cajun seasoning, and breadcrumbs in a large bowl. Mix with a spoon or rubber spatula until well combined.
2. Form the mixture into patties, using approximately ¼ cup of the mixture per patty.
3. In a skillet, heat 3 tablespoons of oil over medium heat.
4. Fry the patties for about 2 minutes on each side or until golden brown. Work in batches if needed. Place the fried croquettes on a plate lined with a paper towel to absorb any excess oil.
5. Squeeze fresh lemon on the croquettes, serve and enjoy.

NOTES:

NICK'S NUTRITIONAL NUGGETS

OMEGA 3 – FATTY ACIDS

1. There are three types of omega-3 fatty acids, alpha-linolenic acid (ALA), eicosapentaenoic acid (EPA), and docosahexaenoic acid (DHA). ALA comes from plant oils, nuts, and seeds like flaxseed oil, walnuts, and chia seeds. EPA and DHA come from fish and seafood.

2. Some research has suggested omega-3 fatty acids (specifically EPA) may assist in the treatment of depression.

3. Omega-3 may assist with blood pressure, brain health, and eye health.

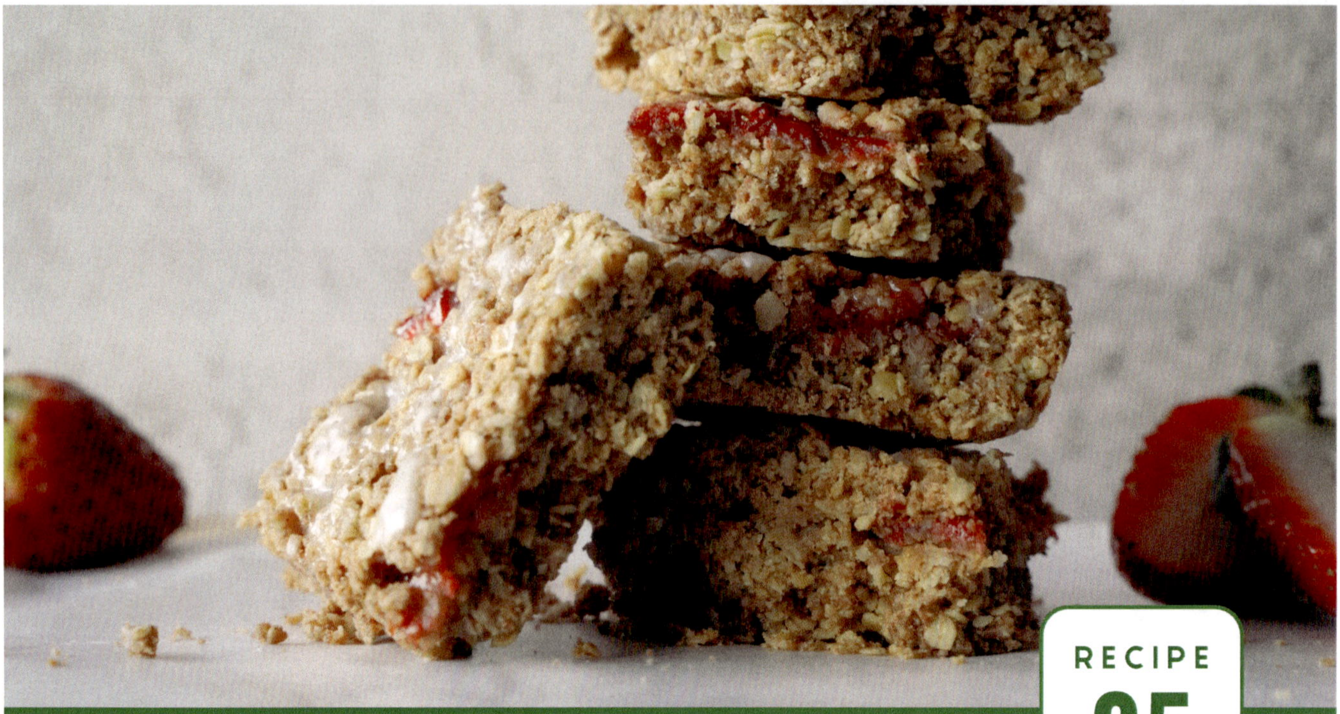

RECIPE 05

SNACKS RECIPES

STRAWBERRY CINNAMON BREAKFAST BARS

INGREDIENTS

BAR

1/2 cup all-purpose flour (62.5g)
1/4 cup dark brown sugar - packed (48g)
2 tablespoons ground cinnamon (15.8g)
1 tablespoon allspice (6g)
1/4 teaspoon salt (1.5g)
1/2 cup cubed unsalted butter (113.5g)
2 cup quick oats (162g)
1 teaspoon vanilla extract (4.2g)
1 tablespoon pulp-free orange juice (15.5g)

PREPARATION

BAR

1. Preheat the oven to 375°F (190°C). Spray 9x9-inch a baking pan with non-stick cooking spray.
2. Put the flour, dark brown sugar, cinnamon, allspice, and salt in a food processor and combine by pulsing several times.
3. Add the cubed butter to the processor. Pulse until the butter has been incorporated into the crumb mixture.
4. Add the oats and pulse to combine again. Remove 1 cup of the mixture and set aside to use for the topping.
5. Add the vanilla extract and orange juice to the processor and pulse to combine.
6. Transfer the mixture onto the greased baking pan. Use your hands to press it into the pan evenly.

INGREDIENTS

FILLING

2 tablespoons dark brown sugar - packed (24g)
1 tablespoon all-purpose flour (7.8g)
2 tablespoons pulp-free orange juice (31g)
1 cup sliced strawberries (166g)

PREPARATION

FILLING :

1. In a medium bowl, add the brown sugar, flour, and orange juice and mix until moistened.
2. Add the sliced strawberries to the brown sugar mixture. Mix until the strawberries are coated. Distribute the strawberries evenly over the dough in the baking pan.
3. Sprinkle the reserved crumb topping evenly over the strawberries.
4. Place a large piece of parchment paper over the mixture and press down very hard with your hands. Smooth along the edges with your fingertips. (This will help the bars hold together). Discard the parchment paper.
5. Spray the top of the bars with non-stick cooking spray.
6. Bake for 40-45 minutes, or until slightly firm and golden brown around the edges. Leave the bars to cool completely before glazing.

INGREDIENTS

GLAZE

1/2 cup powdered sugar - sifted (60g)
1 teaspoon vanilla extract (4.2g)
1/2 teaspoon ground cinnamon (1.3g)
1 tablespoon whole milk (15g)

PREPARATION

GLAZE :

1. In a medium bowl, add the sifted powdered sugar, vanilla and ground cinnamon, and whisk together.
2. Pour the milk into a small cup and warm in the microwave for 15 seconds.
3. Slowly add the milk to the powdered sugar mixture, and whisk often, stopping before each addition, until a drizzle consistency is reached.
4. Once the bars have cooled, drizzle the glaze on top, then cut, serve, and enjoy.

NOTES:

nutrition facts snacks

Sweet Potato Hummus

Nutrition Facts

4 servings per container
Serving size 3.5 oz (0.0g)

Amount Per Serving	
Calories	**460**
	% Daily Value*
Total Fat 31g	**40%**
Saturated Fat 4.5g	**23%**
Trans Fat 0g	
Polyunsaturated Fat 9g	
Monounsaturated Fat 16g	
Cholesterol 0mg	**0%**
Sodium 330mg	**14%**
Total Carbohydrate 37g	**13%**
Dietary Fiber 8g	**29%**
Total Sugars 7g	
Includes 0g Added Sugars	**0%**
Protein 12g	
Vitamin D 0mcg	0%
Calcium 110mg	8%
Iron 4.5mg	25%
Potassium 570mg	10%

* The % Daily Value (DV) tells you how much a nutrient in a serving of food contributes to a daily diet. 2,000 calories a day is used for general nutrition advice.

Sweet & Spicy Guacamole

Nutrition Facts

4 servings per container
Serving size 1/4 cup (0.0g)

Amount Per Serving	
Calories	**410**
	% Daily Value*
Total Fat 34g	**44%**
Saturated Fat 5g	**25%**
Trans Fat 0g	
Cholesterol 0mg	**0%**
Sodium 550mg	**24%**
Total Carbohydrate 31g	**11%**
Dietary Fiber 16g	**57%**
Total Sugars 9g	
Includes 6g Added Sugars	**12%**
Protein 5g	
Vitamin D 0mcg	0%
Calcium 50mg	4%
Iron 1.7mg	10%
Potassium 1230mg	25%

* The % Daily Value (DV) tells you how much a nutrient in a serving of food contributes to a daily diet. 2,000 calories a day is used for general nutrition advice.

Goat Cheese Guacamole

Nutrition Facts

4 servings per container
Serving size 1/4 cup (0.0g)

Amount Per Serving	
Calories	**420**
	% Daily Value*
Total Fat 35g	**45%**
Saturated Fat 6g	**30%**
Trans Fat 0g	
Cholesterol <5mg	**1%**
Sodium 340mg	**15%**
Total Carbohydrate 28g	**10%**
Dietary Fiber 17g	**61%**
Total Sugars 5g	
Includes 0g Added Sugars	**0%**
Protein 7g	
Vitamin D 0mcg	0%
Calcium 60mg	4%
Iron 1.8mg	10%
Potassium 1210mg	25%

* The % Daily Value (DV) tells you how much a nutrient in a serving of food contributes to a daily diet. 2,000 calories a day is used for general nutrition advice.

Cajun Salmon Croquettes

Nutrition Facts

5 servings per container
Serving size 1 cake (0.0g)

Amount Per Serving	
Calories	**420**
	% Daily Value*
Total Fat 30g	**38%**
Saturated Fat 20g	**100%**
Trans Fat 0g	
Cholesterol 140mg	**47%**
Sodium 2480mg	**108%**
Total Carbohydrate 15g	**5%**
Dietary Fiber <1g	**4%**
Total Sugars 5g	
Includes 0g Added Sugars	**0%**
Protein 22g	
Vitamin D 0.5mcg	2%
Calcium 50mg	4%
Iron 2.6mg	15%
Potassium 530mg	10%

* The % Daily Value (DV) tells you how much a nutrient in a serving of food contributes to a daily diet. 2,000 calories a day is used for general nutrition advice.

Strawberry Cinnamon Breakfast Bars

Nutrition Facts

4 servings per container
Serving size 1 - 4x4 square (0.0g)

Amount Per Serving	
Calories	**470**
	% Daily Value*
Total Fat 26g	**33%**
Saturated Fat 15g	**75%**
Trans Fat 1.5g	
Cholesterol 60mg	**20%**
Sodium 150mg	**7%**
Total Carbohydrate 56g	**20%**
Dietary Fiber 7g	**25%**
Total Sugars 22g	
Includes 18g Added Sugars	**36%**
Protein 6g	
Vitamin D 0mcg	0%
Calcium 90mg	6%
Iron 2.4mg	15%
Potassium 280mg	6%

* The % Daily Value (DV) tells you how much a nutrient in a serving of food contributes to a daily diet. 2,000 calories a day is used for general nutrition advice.

In the late 1800's, snacks were considered low-class as they did not require utensils to eat them.

DID YOU KNOW?

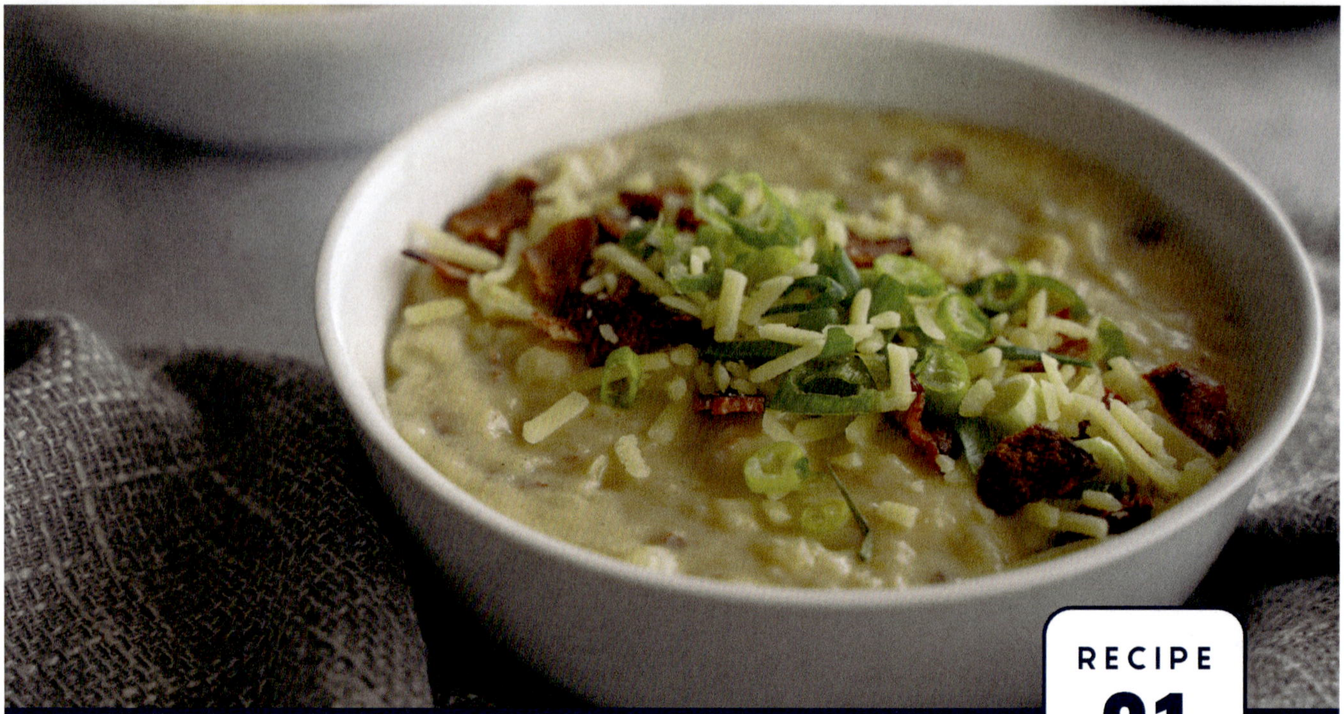

RECIPE 01

LOADED POTATO SOUP

INGREDIENTS

8 peeled and cubed Russet potatoes (1336g)
6 slices thick-cut turkey bacon - or favorite bacon (1/3 cup crumbled, 27.1g)
1/2 cup unsalted butter (113.5g)
1 cup chopped white onion (160g)
1/2 cup chopped green bell pepper (74.5g)
2½ teaspoons minced garlic (12.5g)
1/2 cup all-purpose flour (62.5g)
4 cups whole milk (976g)
1 teaspoon salt (6g)
1/2 teaspoon ground black pepper (1.2g)
1/2 cup shredded cheddar cheese (2.25 oz., 56g)

PREPARATION

1. In a medium pot, bring 8 cups of water to a boil.
2. Place the potatoes in the boiling water and cook for 10 minutes, or until soft.
3. In a medium skillet over medium heat, cook the bacon for 4-7 minutes on each side, or until crispy. When done, transfer to a paper towel-lined plate to drain. Crumble the bacon when cooled.
4. When the potatoes have finished cooking, remove them from the water. Reserve the cooking water in a bowl for later use.
5. In a medium pot over medium-high heat, add the butter, onions, bell peppers and garlic, and cook for 3-5 minutes, or until the butter is melted and the vegetables have softened.
6. Add the flour to the vegetables and stir to combine. Slowly add the reserved potato water and whisk until smooth, then gradually stir in the milk. Cook on medium-high heat for 5 minutes stirring frequently.
7. Add the crumbled bacon, potatoes, salt, and black pepper to the pot, then reduce heat to medium-low, and simmer for 10 minutes.
8. Add the cheddar cheese and mix until melted and well blended. Serve hot.

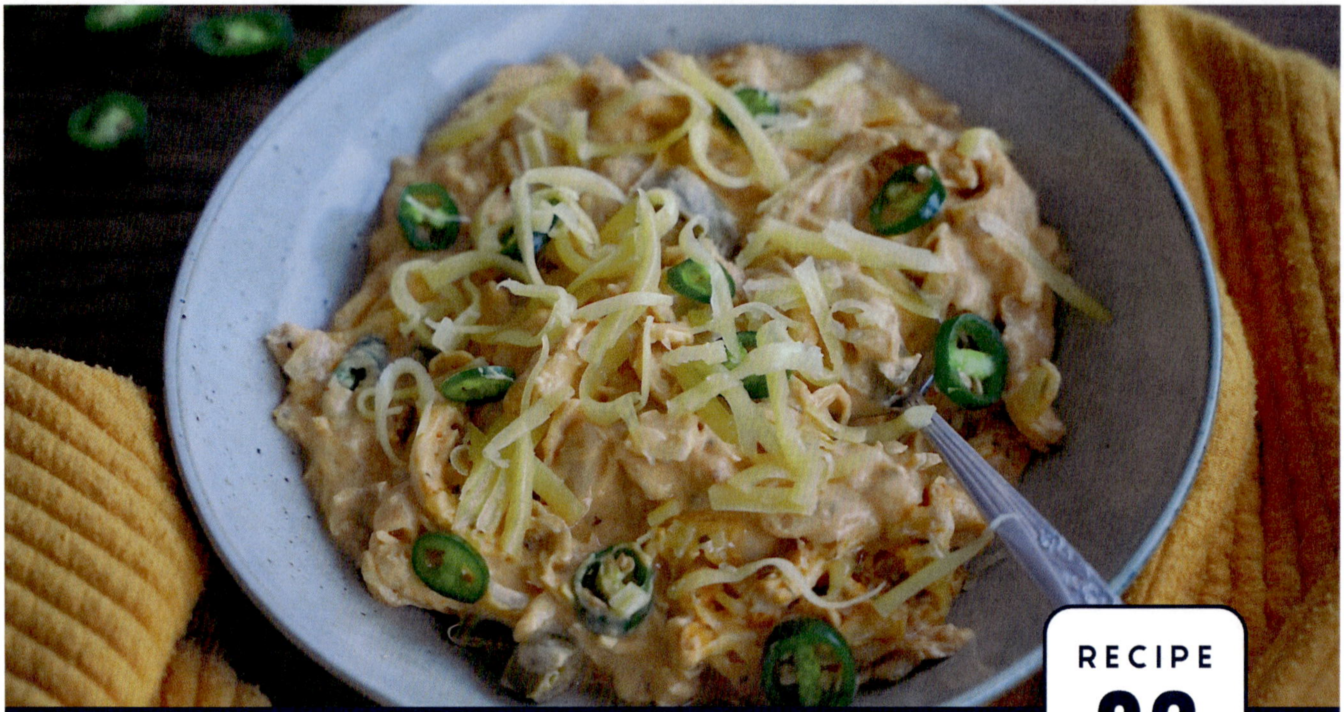

RECIPE 02

BUFFALO CHICKEN DIP CHILI

SOUPS RECIPES

INGREDIENTS

3 chicken breasts (255.2g)
28 oz. low sodium chicken broth (793.8g)
12 oz. cream cheese (340.2g)
1/4 cup whole milk (61g)
1/2 cup Frank's Hot Sauce (4 oz., 113.4g)
1 cup chopped white onion (160g)
4 oz. can green chilies - chopped (113.4g)
1 teaspoon minced garlic (5g)
2 - 14.5 oz. cans Great Northern Beans - drained (822.2g)
2 teaspoons ground cumin (4g)
2 teaspoons dried oregano (3.6g)
1 Packet Ranch Dressing mix (1 oz., 28.4g)
8 oz. shredded Colby & Monterey Jack cheese (224g)

PREPARATION

1. Fill a large saucepan with enough water to cover the chicken breasts. Bring to a boil over medium-high heat and cook the chicken for 20-25 minutes, or until the chicken is tender with no pink present.
2. When the chicken is done, remove it from the water and use two forks to shred it.
3. In another large saucepan, combine the chicken broth, cream cheese, milk, and Frank's hot sauce. Cook on low heat, stirring until creamy and thoroughly combined.
4. Add the shredded chicken, onions, green chilies, garlic, beans, ground cumin, dried oregano, ranch dressing packet, and half of the Colby Monterrey Jack to the saucepan with the chicken broth mixture.
5. Simmer for 20-30 minutes, stirring regularly. Serve hot with the remaining cheese as a topping.

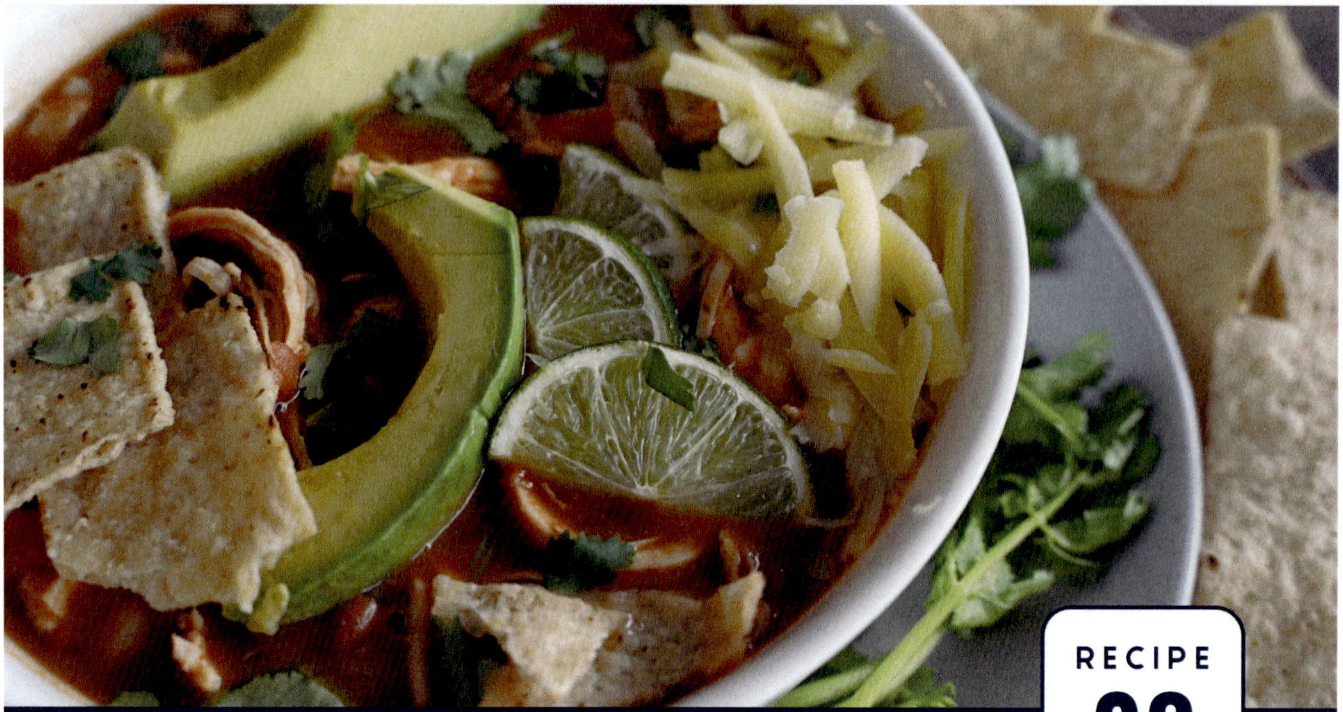

RECIPE
03

CHICKEN TORTILLA SOUP

SOUPS RECIPES

INGREDIENTS

3 chicken breasts (255.2g)
2 tablespoons vegetable oil (27.2g)
1/2 cup diced white onion (80g)
1 tablespoon minced garlic (15g)
1½ tablespoons diced jalapenos (8.4g)
6 cups low-sodium chicken broth (1440g)
14 oz. can fire-roasted diced tomatoes (411.1g)
14.5 oz. can vegetarian refried beans (411.1g)
14.5 oz. can black beans - rinsed and drained (411.1g)
1 teaspoon salt (6g)
1 teaspoon black pepper (2.3g)
2 Limes - 1 for juice and 1 for garnish (134g)
1 cup chopped fresh cilantro leaves (16g)
1 oz. tri-colored tortilla strips (7-10 strips, 28.4g)
1 cup chopped avocado (146g)
4 oz. shredded Colby & Monterrey Jack cheese (112g)

PREPARATION

1. Fill a large saucepan with enough water to cover the chicken breasts. Bring to a boil over medium-high heat, cook the chicken for 20-25 minutes, or until the chicken is tender with no pink present.
2. When the chicken is done, remove it from the water and use two forks to shred it.
3. In another large saucepan, heat the vegetable oil over medium heat. Add the onions and cook for 2 minutes. Once the onions have softened, add the garlic and jalapenos and cook for another minute.
4. Add the chicken broth, tomatoes, beans, salt and black pepper to vegetable mix, and bring to a boil.
5. Once at a boil, add the shredded chicken, then reduce to medium-low heat, and simmer for 15 minutes. Add the lime juice and fresh cilantro to the pot.
6. Ladle the soup into serving bowls and top with a lime wedge, tri-colored tortilla strips, avocado slices, and cheese. Serve immediately.

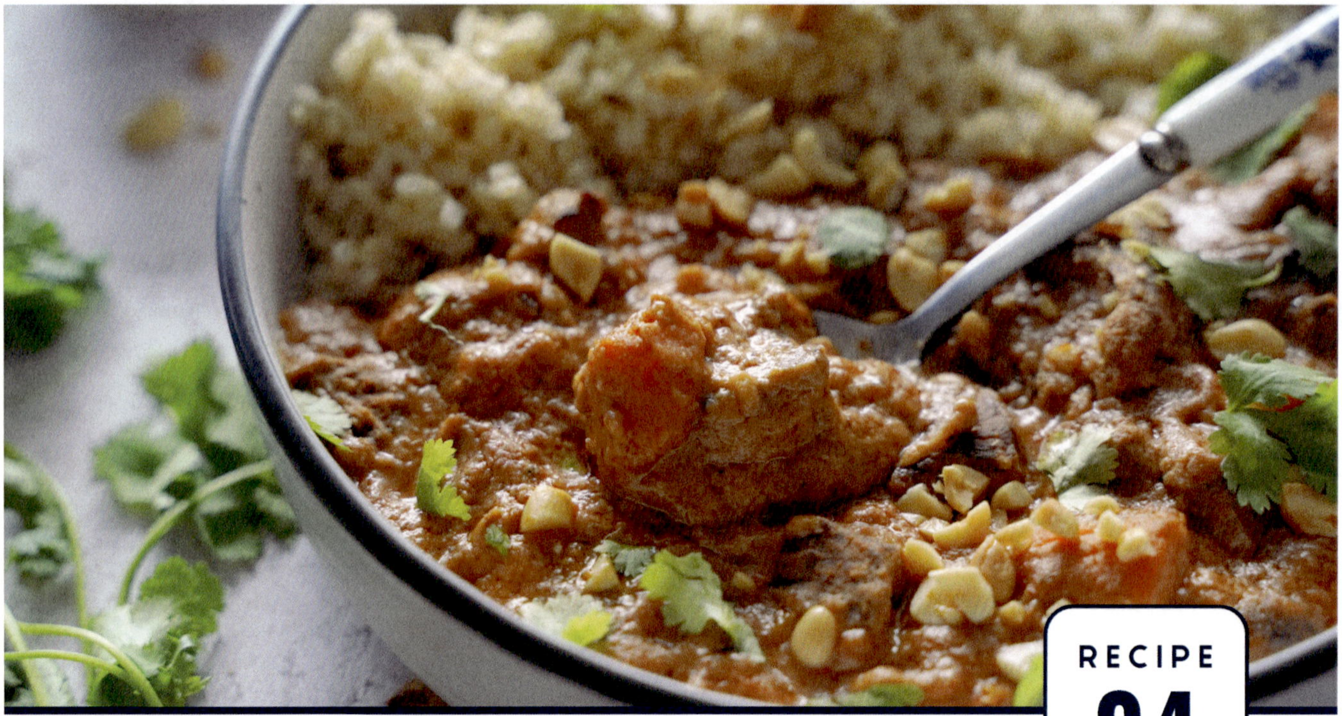

RECIPE 04

PEANUT BUTTER STEW

INGREDIENTS

RICE

1 cup long grain white rice (185g)
2 cups water (474g)
Pinch of salt

PREPARATION

RICE

1. In a fine strainer, rinse rice under cold water until the water runs clear.
2. In a medium saucepan over medium heat, bring the water to a boil. Add rice and salt.
3. Bring to a low boil, then lower heat, cover the saucepan and cook covered for 18 minutes, or until the rice is tender and all the water is absorbed.
4. Turn off the heat, strain the rice to remove excess liquid, if any, and then set aside for 5 minutes. Fluff with a fork, and then set aside.

INGREDIENTS

STEW

3 cups water (711g)
1/2 pound beef chunks (8 oz., 226.8g)
1/2 teaspoon salt (3g)
1/2 teaspoon black pepper (1.2g)
1½ tablespoons all-purpose seasoning (18g)
1/2 teaspoon onion powder (1.2g)
1/2 teaspoon crushed red pepper flakes (1g)
1 beef bouillon cube (3.6g)
1 tablespoon vegetable oil (13.6g)
1/2 cup chopped red onion (88.8g)
1 teaspoon minced garlic (5g)
1/2 cup cubed sweet potatoes (66.5g)
8 oz. canned tomatoes - chopped with liquid (226.8g)
1/2 cup smooth no salt added peanut butter (129g)

PREPARATION

STEW

1. In a large pot, heat the water over medium-high heat.
2. Season the beef chunks with salt, black pepper, all-purpose seasoning, onion powder, and crushed red pepper flakes. In a large skillet on medium heat add the beef and cook for 15-20 minutes or until tender and cooked through, set beef aside.
3. Once the water is hot, add the beef bouillon cube into water and cook for about 10 minutes, once the cube has dissolved; add the cooked beef chunks to the water, and cook for another 5 minutes.
4. Remove the beef from the water, set aside and reserve the cooking water.
5. In another large skillet, heat the vegetable oil over medium-high heat. Add the onion and garlic, then cook, stirring often for 5 minutes, or until softened.
6. Lower the heat under the vegetable skillet to medium heat and add the beef chunks. Cook, stirring occasionally, for 5 minutes.
7. Place the sweet potatoes in the beef cooking water and bring to a boil over medium-high heat.
8. Reduce heat to low and cover the pot partially with a lid. Simmer for 15 minutes.
9. Add the beef vegetable mixture, tomatoes, and peanut butter to the pot and combine. Partially cover the pot again and continue cooking, stirring occasionally, for another 20 minutes.
10. Ladle the soup over cooked rice in a serving bowl. Serve immediately and enjoy.

NICK'S NUTRITIONAL NUGGETS

Peanut stew is called maafe, it's a staple food in Western Africa. It originates from the Mandinka and Bambara people of Mali.

nutrition facts soups

Loaded Potato Soup

Nutrition Facts

5 servings per container
Serving size 8 oz (0.0g)

Amount Per Serving	
Calories	**640**
	% Daily Value*
Total Fat 30g	**38%**
Saturated Fat 18g	**90%**
Trans Fat 1g	
Cholesterol 85mg	**28%**
Sodium 760mg	**33%**
Total Carbohydrate 78g	**28%**
Dietary Fiber 6g	**21%**
Total Sugars 14g	
Includes 0g Added Sugars	**0%**
Protein 17g	
Vitamin D 0.1mcg	0%
Calcium 340mg	25%
Iron 1.7mg	10%
Potassium 1260mg	25%

* The % Daily Value (DV) tells you how much a nutrient in a serving of food contributes to a daily diet. 2,000 calories a day is used for general nutrition advice.

Buffalo Chicken Dip Chili

Nutrition Facts

6 servings per container
Serving size 8 oz (0.0g)

Amount Per Serving	
Calories	**600**
	% Daily Value*
Total Fat 34g	**44%**
Saturated Fat 19g	**95%**
Trans Fat 0.5g	
Cholesterol 125mg	**42%**
Sodium 1960mg	**85%**
Total Carbohydrate 40g	**15%**
Dietary Fiber 11g	**39%**
Total Sugars 5g	
Includes 0g Added Sugars	**0%**
Protein 38g	
Vitamin D 0mcg	0%
Calcium 540mg	40%
Iron 4.5mg	25%
Potassium 880mg	20%

* The % Daily Value (DV) tells you how much a nutrient in a serving of food contributes to a daily diet. 2,000 calories a day is used for general nutrition advice.

Chicken Tortilla Soup

Nutrition Facts

6 servings per container
Serving size 8 oz (0.0g)

Amount Per Serving	
Calories	**440**
	% Daily Value*
Total Fat 18g	**23%**
Saturated Fat 8g	**40%**
Trans Fat 0g	
Cholesterol 45mg	**15%**
Sodium 1110mg	**48%**
Total Carbohydrate 42g	**15%**
Dietary Fiber 12g	**43%**
Total Sugars 4g	
Includes 0g Added Sugars	**0%**
Protein 30g	
Vitamin D 0mcg	0%
Calcium 280mg	20%
Iron 4mg	20%
Potassium 900mg	20%

* The % Daily Value (DV) tells you how much a nutrient in a serving of food contributes to a daily diet. 2,000 calories a day is used for general nutrition advice.

Peanut Butter Stew

Nutrition Facts

About 3 servings per container
Serving size 1 bowl (0.0g)

Amount Per Serving	
Calories	**680**
	% Daily Value*
Total Fat 31g	**40%**
Saturated Fat 10g	**50%**
Trans Fat 0g	
Cholesterol 50mg	**17%**
Sodium 2720mg	**118%**
Total Carbohydrate 72g	**26%**
Dietary Fiber 6g	**21%**
Total Sugars 10g	
Includes 1g Added Sugars	**2%**
Protein 32g	
Vitamin D 0.1mcg	0%
Calcium 100mg	8%
Iron 6.2mg	35%
Potassium 910mg	20%

* The % Daily Value (DV) tells you how much a nutrient in a serving of food contributes to a daily diet. 2,000 calories a day is used for general nutrition advice.

The earliest archaeological evidence for the consumption of soup dates back to 6000 BC, and it was hippopotamus soup.

DID YOU KNOW?

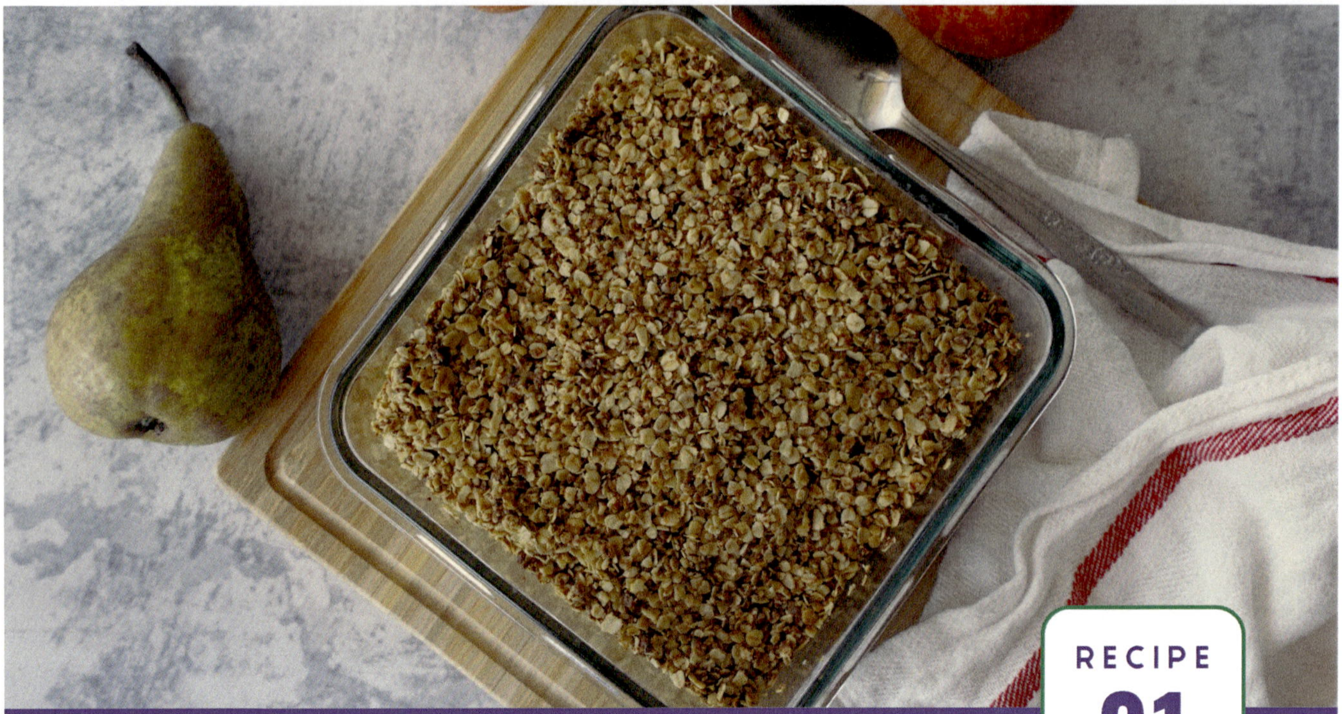

RECIPE 01

APPLE PEAR CRISP

INGREDIENTS

FILLING

3/4 teaspoon cinnamon (2g)

2 tablespoons granulated sugar (25.2g)

1 tablespoon all-purpose flour (14.2g)

2 medium baking apples - cored and sliced thin (322g) (i.e., Granny Smith)

1 medium pear - cored and sliced thin (178g) (i.e., Beurre Bosc)

INGREDIENTS

TOPPING

1 tablespoon all-purpose flour (14.2g)

3/4 teaspoon cinnamon (2g)

1 cup quick oats (49g)

1 teaspoon vanilla extract (4.2g)

1/4 cup light brown sugar - packed (36.3g)

2 tablespoons unsalted butter (28.4g), at room temperature

1 tablespoon caramel syrup - drizzle (40g)

PREPARATION

FILLING:

1. Preheat the oven to 325°F (160°C).
2. Spray an 8x8-inch baking dish with non-stick cooking spray and set aside.
3. In a medium bowl, combine the cinnamon, granulated sugar and flour using a fork.
4. Add the sliced apples and pears to the cinnamon mixture, and toss until the fruit pieces are evenly coated with the cinnamon mixture. Transfer the mixture to the baking dish and spread evenly over the dish.

TOPPING:

1. To make the topping, combine the flour, cinnamon, oats, vanilla, brown sugar, butter and mix with a fork until crumbly.
2. Sprinkle the topping evenly over the fruit in the baking dish.
3. Bake for 25 minutes, or until the apples are soft and the topping is golden brown.
4. Drizzle the caramel syrup over the fruit topping mixture
5. Cool for 10 minutes before serving.

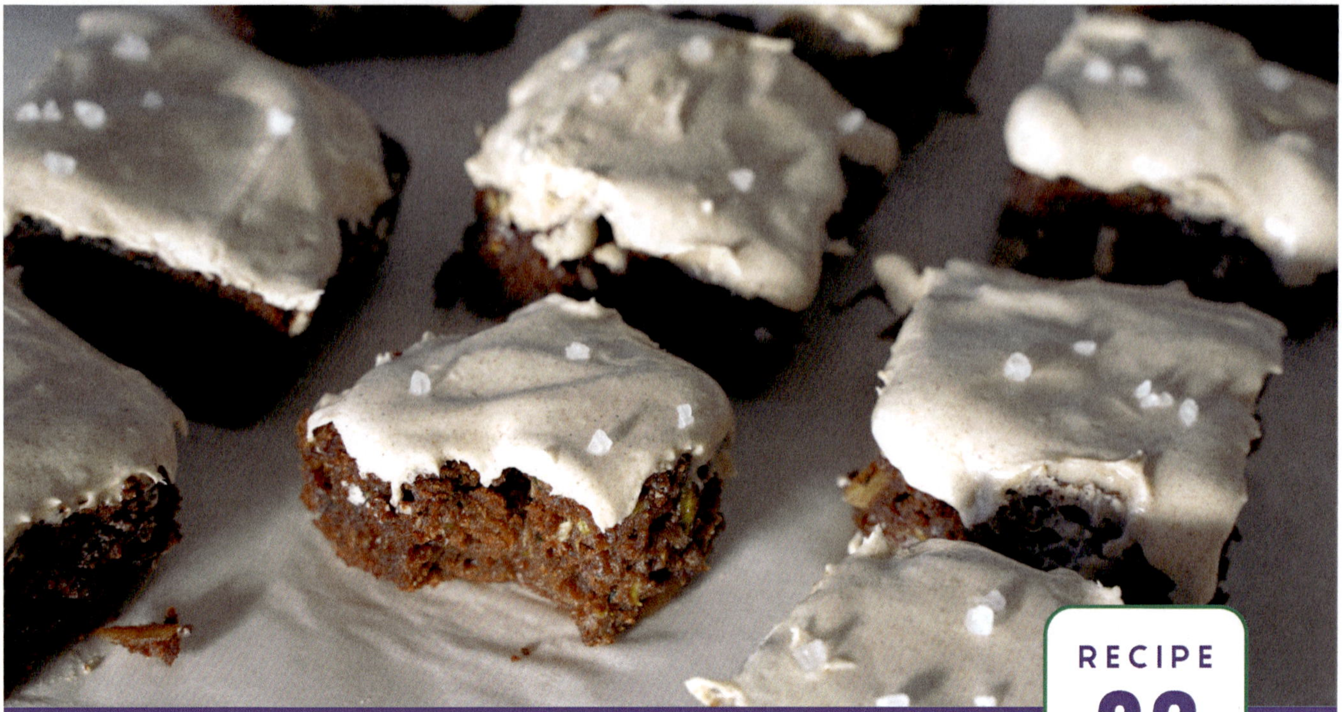

RECIPE 02

ZUCCHINI-ALMOND BROWNIES WITH CREAM TOPPING

INGREDIENTS

BROWNIE

1/2 cup vegetable oil (109g)
1/4 cup unsweetened applesauce (56.7g) [or 1 jumbo egg (63g)]
1½ cups granulated sugar (300g)
2 teaspoons vanilla extract (8.4g)
2 cups all-purpose flour (250g)
1/2 cup unsweetened cocoa powder (43g)
2 teaspoons baking soda (9.2g)
1¾ cups grated, undrained zucchini (396.9g)
1/2 cup sliced almonds (46g)

PREPARATION

BROWNIE:

1. Preheat the oven to 350°F (175°C).
2. Lightly grease a 13x9-inch baking dish with non-stick cooking spray. Lightly dust the greased pan with flour.
3. Add the oil, applesauce or egg, sugar, and vanilla in a large bowl. Whisk until well blended.
4. In a separate bowl, add the flour, cocoa powder, baking soda and briefly whisk to combine.

5. Add the flour mixture to the sugar mixture and stir well with a wooden spoon or rubber spatula until thoroughly mixed. (It will appear quite dry)
6. Gently fold in the zucchini and almonds. Spread the batter evenly into the prepared baking dish.
7. Bake for 30-40 minutes, or until a toothpick inserted in the center of the brownies comes out clean. Allow the brownies to completely cool before frosting.

INGREDIENTS

FROSTING

6 tablespoons Kraft Marshmallow Cream (3 oz., 85g)
7 tablespoons cream cheese (3.5 oz., 99.2g), at room temperature
1/4 cup heavy whipping cream (59.2g)
1 teaspoon cinnamon (2.6g)

PREPARATION

FROSTING:

1. While the brownies are cooling, add the marshmallow cream, cream cheese, heavy cream, and cinnamon in a medium bowl and mix until smooth.
2. Spread the frosting evenly over the cooled brownies. Cut the brownies, serve and enjoy.

NICK'S NUTRITIONAL NUGGETS

Applesauce can be used as a substitute for various baking ingredients. For example eggs and butter.

BUTTER

i. Applesauce can help act as a binding agent when baking. *Although it can create a slight change in taste and texture*
ii. Replace applesauce with approximately half of the amount of butter needed.

EGGS

i. The ability to replace eggs is primarily due to the pectin in applesauce.
ii. Eggs prevent the gluten in flour to become networks; pectin polysaccharides have the same effect on the gluten in flour.

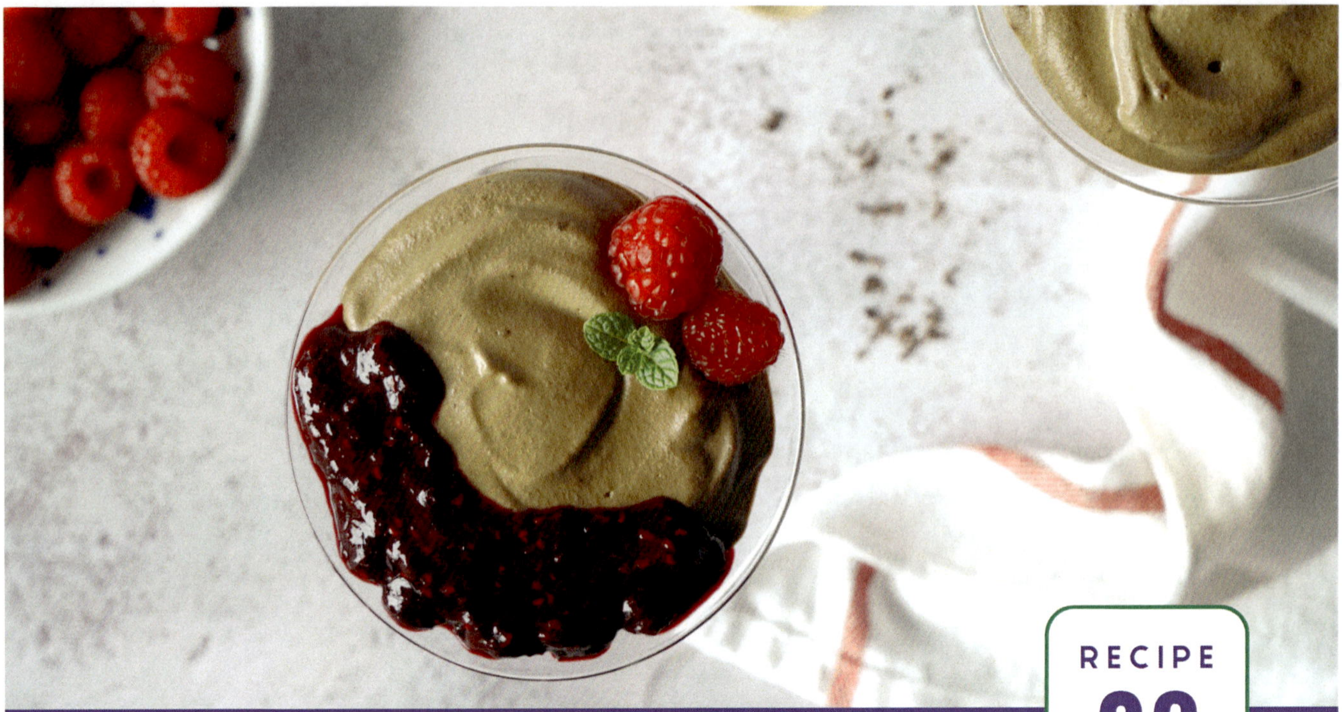

RECIPE 03

CHOCOLATE MOUSSE WITH FRUIT PRESERVE TOPPING

INGREDIENTS

CHOCOLATE MOUSSE

2/3 cup smashed ripe avocado (154.1g)

1/4 cup honey or 1/4 cup maple syrup (84.8g) [1/4 cup granulated sugar (50g)]

1/2 cup regular unsweetened coconut milk (4 oz., 113.4g)

1 teaspoon vanilla extract (4.2g)

1/3 cup dark chocolate chips (53.3g) [or dark cocoa powder 1/4 cup (24g)

PREPARATION

CHOCOLATE MOUSS:

1. Place the avocado, honey or maple syrup, coconut milk, and vanilla in a blender and pulse until smooth.
   a. *Alternate* Place avocado, granulated sugar, dark cocoa powder, coconut milk, and vanilla in a blender and pulse until smooth ***Then skip to step 4***
2. In a small saucepan over medium-low heat, melt chocolate chips. Stir frequently to ensure the chocolate does not burn. Once melted, remove from the heat and leave to cool completely.
3. In a medium bowl, combine the avocado mixture and the melted chocolate chips and stir until smooth.
4. Refrigerate the mousse for at least 1 hour before serving.

DESSERT RECIPES

INGREDIENTS

FRUIT PRESERVES

2 cups frozen mixed berries (280g)
1/2 cup granulated sugar (100g)
2 tablespoons lemon juice (1 oz., 28.4g)
Pinch of salt

PREPARATION

FRUITS PRESERVES

1. In a medium saucepan over medium heat, add mixed berries, sugar, lemon juice and a pinch of salt. Stir often to ensure fruit does not burn, cook until the sugar dissolves and the fruit is tender and well blended. ***Do NOT Boil***
2. Reduce the heat to low and gently simmer for 10 minutes, or until the jam is set. The jam should be semi-solid and thick, not runny (i.e. cold plate test).
3. Remove from the heat. For short-term storage, completely cool the preserves and store in an air-tight container in the refrigerator for up to two weeks. For longer-term storage, pour the hot preserves into a sterilized jam jar. Follow water bath canning instructions (https://nchfp.uga.edu/publications/uga/using_bw_canners.html) and store at room temperature.
4. When ready to serve, remove chocolate mousse from the refrigerator and top with the cooled preserves. Serve and enjoy.

NICK'S NUTRITIONAL NUGGETS

Dark chocolate is rich in antioxidants. Antioxidants scavenge free radicals from the body's cells and prevent or reduce the damage caused by oxidation.

Free radicals are single atoms that naturally occur in the body, that run amuck looking for a partner, causing damage to cells, proteins, and DNA.

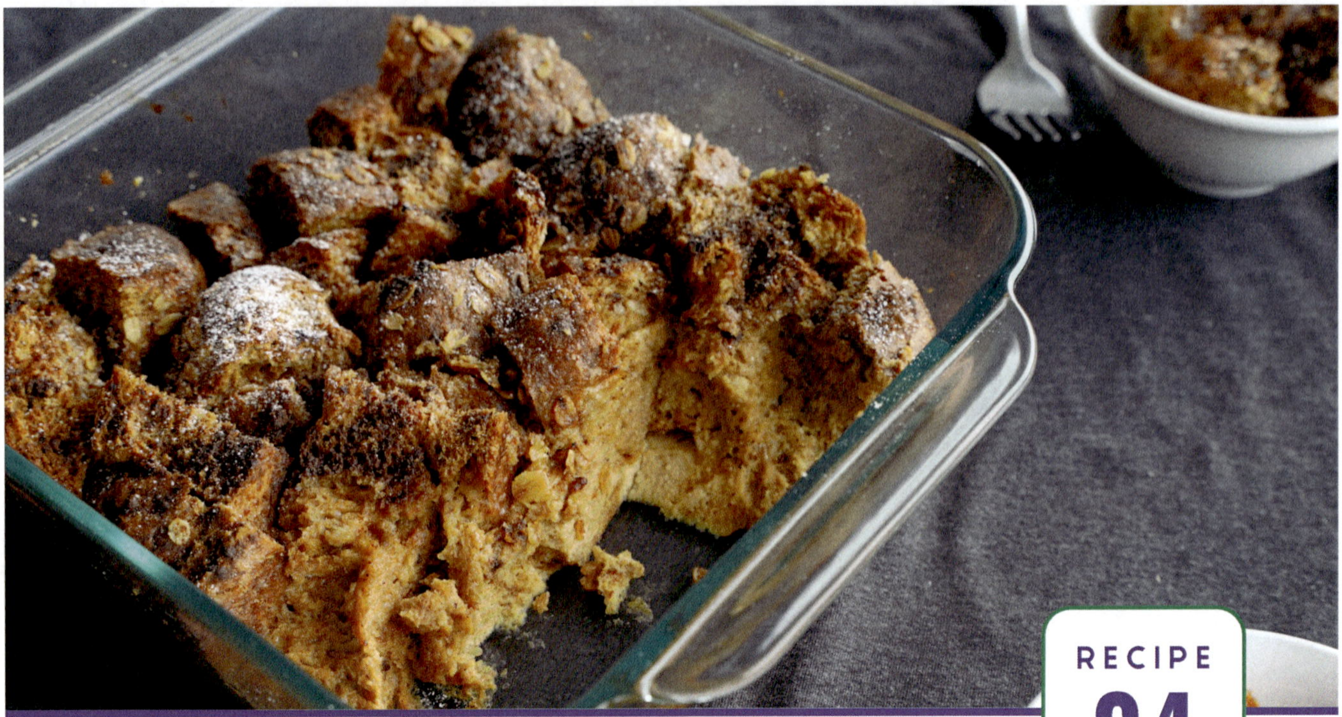

RECIPE 04

SMOKED CHIPOTLE MAPLE SYRUP BREAD PUDDING

INGREDIENTS

1/4 cup butter (56.8g)
1/2 loaf bread - stale or fresh (8 slices, 200g)
4 jumbo eggs (252g)
1/4 cup light brown sugar - packed (36.3g)
1 teaspoon vanilla extract (4.2g)
1 teaspoon cinnamon (2.6g)
1 cup evaporated milk (252g)
1/2 cup whole milk (122g)
1/3 cup maple syrup (2.67 oz., 75.7g)
1 tablespoon chipotle pepper powder (3g)

DESSERT RECIPES

PREPARATION

1. Melt the butter in the microwave (be sure to cover it with a plate or paper towel) or in a small pan on the stove.
2. Cut the slices of bread into cubes.
3. Place the eggs, brown sugar, vanilla, 1/2 a teaspoon of cinnamon, evaporated milk, and whole milk in a large mixing bowl and mix well with a whisk.
4. Lightly grease an 8x8-inch aluminum pan or casserole-baking dish with non-sticking cooking spray.
5. Transfer the bread cubes to the pan and pour half of the melted butter over the bread.
6. In another large bowl, add the maple syrup, chipotle pepper, and remaining butter; mix until smooth.
7. Pour the brown sugar mixture (step 3) and chipotle mixture (step 6) over the bread, making sure it is evenly coated. Cover the baking dish with plastic wrap or foil and transfer to the refrigerator. Allow the bread to soak for at least 1 hour, and preferably overnight.
8. Preheat the oven to 350°F (175°C).
9. Sprinkle the remaining 1/2 teaspoon of cinnamon over the top of the bread mixture.
10. Bake for 1 hour, or until the top is lightly browned and the center has set. Cool for 10 minutes before serving.

*Note: *If using fresh bread but desire stale bread leave the pieces out overnight, uncovered, to dry the bread cubes out.**

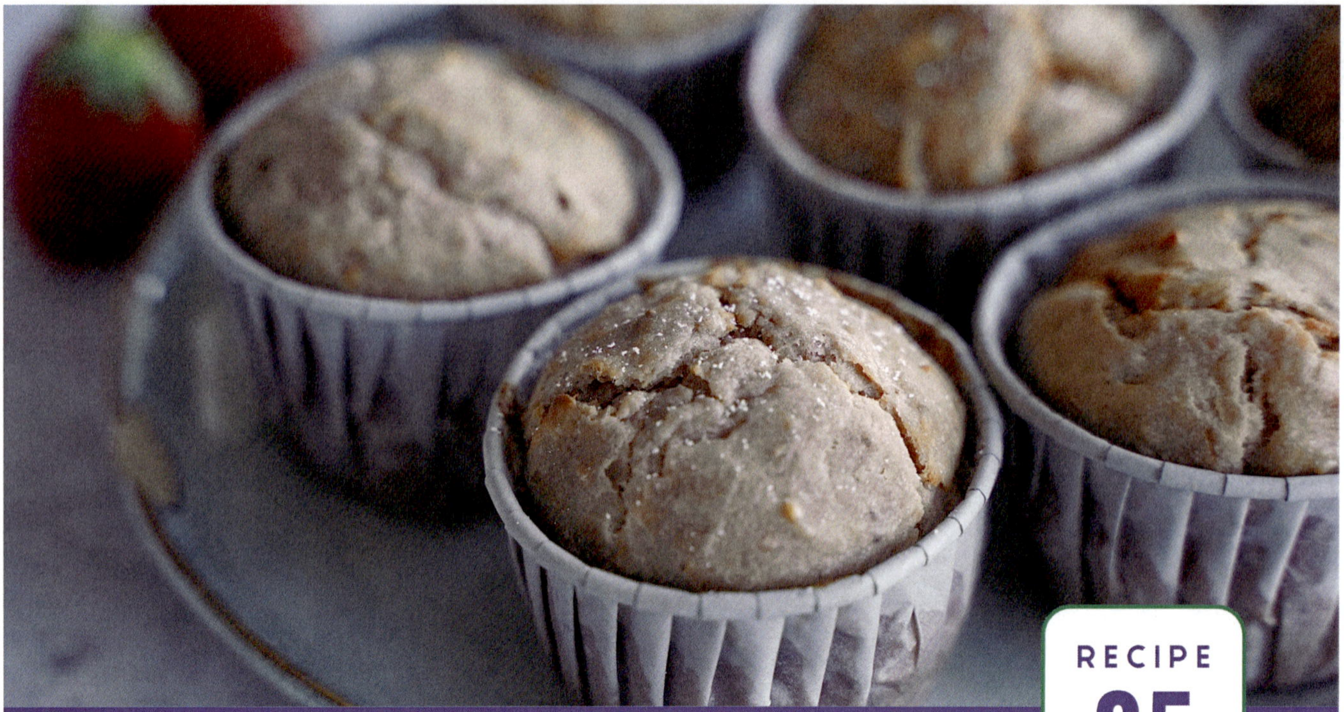

RECIPE 05

STRAWBERRY BANANA CHEESECAKE MUFFINS

INGREDIENTS

1/3 cup mashed banana (74.3g)
2 cups sliced strawberries (332g)
2 cups all-purpose flour (250g)
1½ cups granulated sugar (300g)
1/2 teaspoon baking soda (2.3g)
1 teaspoon salt (6g)
1 teaspoon vanilla extract (4.2g)
1/4 cup butter (56.8g), at room temperature
2 large eggs (126g), at room temperature
3/4 cup cream cheese (6 oz., 174g), at room temperature

PREPARATION

1. Preheat the oven to 425°F (220°C).
2. Line a muffin tin with baking cup liners, or grease lightly with non-stick cooking spray.
3. Place the mashed bananas and strawberries into a blender and pulse 3 times for 30 seconds each, or until fully pureed.
4. In a medium bowl, whisk together the flour, sugar, baking powder, and salt.
5. In a separate bowl, beat together the vanilla, butter, eggs, cream cheese, and strawberry-banana puree. Be sure to mix thoroughly; once the dry ingredients are added, be careful to not over-mix.
6. Add the dry ingredients to the wet ingredients, stir gently with a fork, or fold together with a spatula.
7. Fill the muffin cups about three-quarters of the way up.
8. Bake the muffins for 20 minutes, or until golden brown on the top, and a toothpick inserted in the center comes out clean.
9. Remove muffins from the oven and cool in the pan for 10 minutes, then carefully remove the muffins from the tin and transfer them to a wire rack to cool.

*Note: *Do not leave the muffins in the pan for too long, or the residual heat will continue to cook them.**

nutrition facts desserts

Apple Pear Crisp

Nutrition Facts

1 serving per container
Serving size **1 bowl (6 oz) (0.0g)**

Amount Per Serving	
Calories	**550**
	% Daily Value*
Total Fat 13g	**17%**
Saturated Fat 8g	**40%**
Trans Fat 0.5g	
Cholesterol 30mg	**10%**
Sodium 200mg	**9%**
Total Carbohydrate 109g	**40%**
Dietary Fiber 8g	**29%**
Total Sugars 71g	
Includes 45g Added Sugars	**90%**
Protein 5g	
Vitamin D 0mcg	0%
Calcium 150mg	10%
Iron 5.8mg	30%
Potassium 360mg	8%

* The % Daily Value (DV) tells you how much a nutrient in a serving of food contributes to a daily diet. 2,000 calories a day is used for general nutrition advice.

Zucchini-Almond Brownies with Cream Topping

Nutrition Facts

6 servings per container
Serving size **4 x 4 inch square (0.0g)**

Amount Per Serving	
Calories	**720**
	% Daily Value*
Total Fat 32g	**41%**
Saturated Fat 21g	**105%**
Trans Fat 0g	
Cholesterol 60mg	**20%**
Sodium 290mg	**13%**
Total Carbohydrate 104g	**38%**
Dietary Fiber 6g	**21%**
Total Sugars 61g	
Includes 57g Added Sugars	**114%**
Protein 12g	
Vitamin D 0.3mcg	2%
Calcium 80mg	6%
Iron 4mg	20%
Potassium 570mg	10%

* The % Daily Value (DV) tells you how much a nutrient in a serving of food contributes to a daily diet. 2,000 calories a day is used for general nutrition advice.

Chocolate Mousse with Fruit Preserve Topping

Nutrition Facts

About 3 servings per container
Serving size **1 cup (0.0g)**

Amount Per Serving	
Calories	**450**
	% Daily Value*
Total Fat 15g	**19%**
Saturated Fat 6g	**30%**
Trans Fat 0g	
Cholesterol 0mg	**0%**
Sodium 75mg	**3%**
Total Carbohydrate 78g	**28%**
Dietary Fiber 10g	**36%**
Total Sugars 64g	
Includes 56g Added Sugars	**112%**
Protein 4g	
Vitamin D 0mcg	0%
Calcium 20mg	2%
Iron 3.9mg	20%
Potassium 280mg	6%

* The % Daily Value (DV) tells you how much a nutrient in a serving of food contributes to a daily diet. 2,000 calories a day is used for general nutrition advice.

Smoked Chipotle Maple Syrup Bread Pudding

Nutrition Facts

6 servings per container
Serving size **1 cup (0.0g)**

Amount Per Serving	
Calories	**350**
	% Daily Value*
Total Fat 17g	**22%**
Saturated Fat 9g	**45%**
Trans Fat 0g	
Cholesterol 190mg	**63%**
Sodium 280mg	**12%**
Total Carbohydrate 37g	**13%**
Dietary Fiber 1g	**4%**
Total Sugars 21g	
Includes 13g Added Sugars	**26%**
Protein 12g	
Vitamin D 0.9mcg	4%
Calcium 230mg	20%
Iron 2.1mg	10%
Potassium 300mg	6%

* The % Daily Value (DV) tells you how much a nutrient in a serving of food contributes to a daily diet. 2,000 calories a day is used for general nutrition advice.

Strawberry Banana Cheesecake Muffins

Nutrition Facts

8 servings per container
Serving size **1 muffin (0.0g)**

Amount Per Serving	
Calories	**430**
	% Daily Value*
Total Fat 15g	**19%**
Saturated Fat 9g	**45%**
Trans Fat 0g	
Polyunsaturated Fat 1g	
Monounsaturated Fat 4g	
Cholesterol 95mg	**32%**
Sodium 460mg	**20%**
Total Carbohydrate 68g	**25%**
Dietary Fiber 2g	**7%**
Total Sugars 42g	
Includes 37g Added Sugars	**74%**
Protein 7g	
Vitamin D 0.3mcg	2%
Calcium 40mg	4%
Iron 2mg	10%
Potassium 180mg	4%

* The % Daily Value (DV) tells you how much a nutrient in a serving of food contributes to a daily diet. 2,000 calories a day is used for general nutrition advice.

Each year, seven billion chocolate chips are consumed in the United States. This equates to over 19.2 million cookies eaten a day; of this, 50% are still homemade.

DID YOU KNOW?

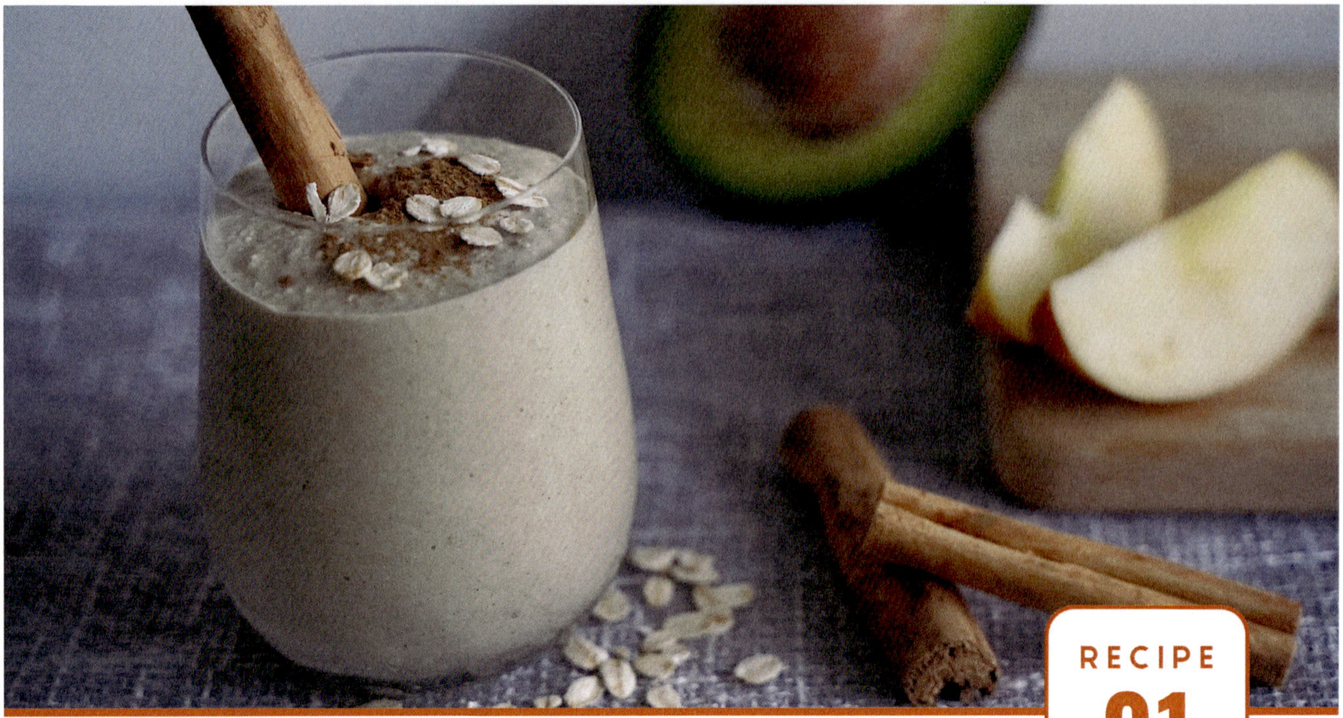

RECIPE 01

APPLE PIE

INGREDIENTS

1/2 ripe avocado - pitted (100.5g)
1 cup whole milk (244g)
1 cup apple butter (256g)
1½ cups quick oats (120g)
1 teaspoon cinnamon (2.6g)
1 teaspoon vanilla extract (4.2g)

PREPARATION

1. Cut the avocado in half and remove the pit. Scoop the flesh into a blender.
2. Pour milk over the avocado and add the apple butter, oatmeal, cinnamon, and vanilla.
3. Blend the mixture on high for about 1 minute or until smooth. The mixture should be a thin enough consistency to drink through a straw. Add additional milk to adjust the consistency if required.
4. Taste the mixture. If it is not sweet enough, add apple butter, or 1 teaspoon honey, or another sweetener, blend for 10-15 seconds and taste.
5. When the mixture has reached the proper consistency and flavor, pour into a large cup and enjoy.

NOTES:

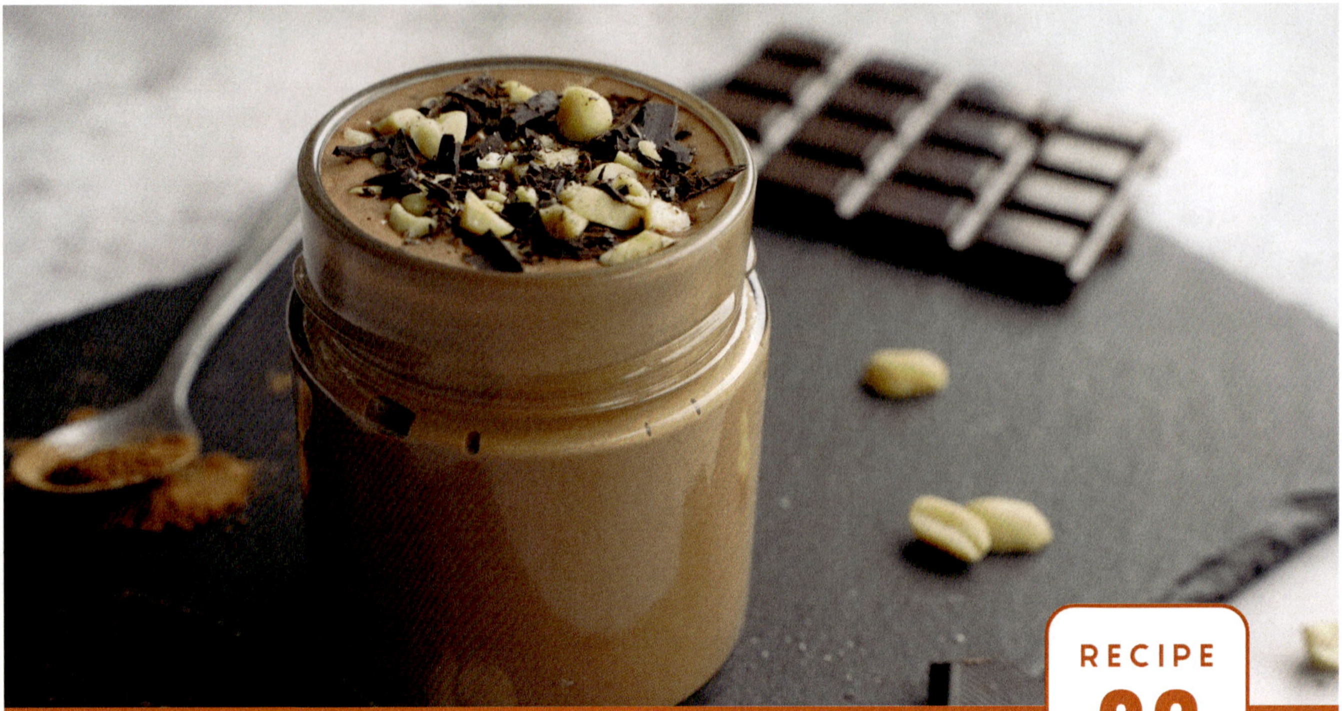

RECIPE 02

THICK AND SWEET

INGREDIENTS

1/2 cup rolled oats (40.5g)
1/2 cup water (118.5g)
4 oz. Greek yogurt (1/2 cup, or 113.4g)
2 tablespoons creamy peanut butter (32g)
1 tablespoon honey (21g)
2 tablespoons unsweetened cocoa powder (10.8g)

PREPARATION

1. Combine the rolled oats and water in a blender and blend on high until completely smooth and creamy.
2. Add the yogurt, peanut butter, honey, and cocoa powder to the oat milk and blend on high for 1 minute, or until smooth. The consistency should be thin enough to drink through a straw. Add additional water to adjust the consistency if required.
3. Taste the mixture. If it is not sweet enough, add 1 teaspoon honey or another sweetener, blend for 10-15 seconds and taste.
4. When the mixture has reached the proper taste and consistency, pour into a large cup and enjoy.

NOTES:

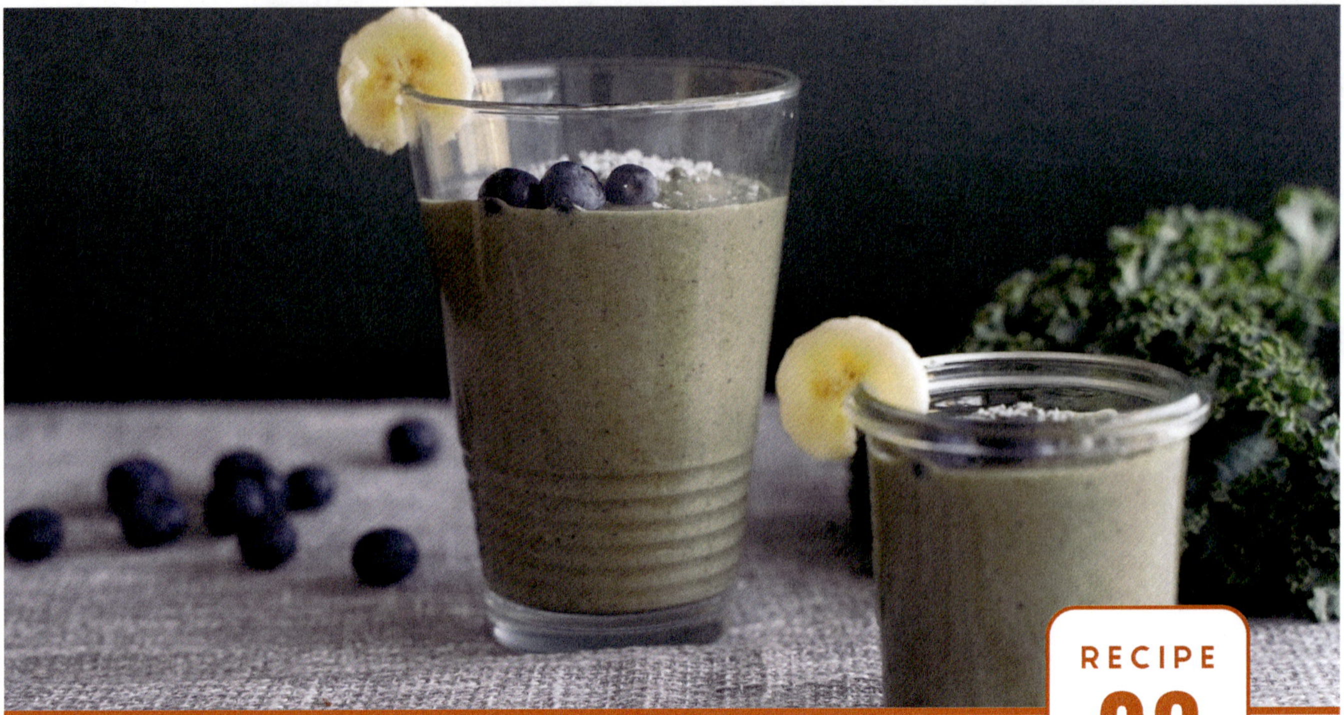

RECIPE
03

MEAN GREEN

INGREDIENTS

1/2 cup rolled oats (40.5g)
3/4 cup water (177.8g)
1/2 avocado - pitted and skin removed (100.5g)
1/2 cup dates - pitted (about 4 oz.,
or 4 large dates (113.4g),
[*Can substitute 1/4 cup honey (84.8g)]
2 tablespoons coconut milk (1 oz., 28.4g)
1 medium banana - peel removed (118g)
1 cup roughly chopped kale (67g)
1/2 cup blueberries (74g)

PREPARATION

1. Combine the rolled oats and water in a blender, and blend on high until completely smooth and creamy.
2. Add the avocado, dates, coconut milk, banana, kale, and blueberries to the blender and blend on high for 1 minute, or until smooth. The consistency should be thin enough to drink through a straw. Add additional water to adjust the consistency if required.
3. Taste the mixture. If it is not sweet enough, add 3 dates or 1 teaspoon of honey, or another sweetener, blend for 10-15 seconds and taste.
4. When the mixture has reached the proper taste and consistency, pour into a large cup and enjoy.

NOTES:

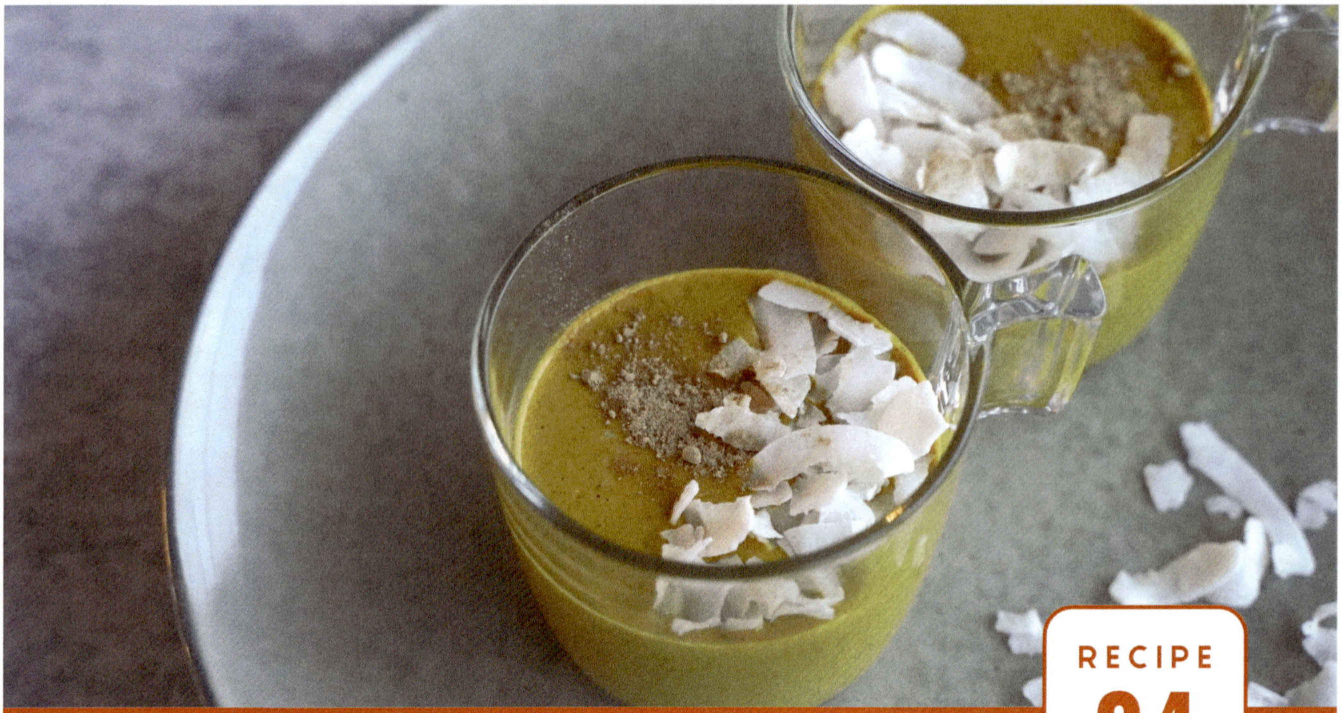

RECIPE 04

GOLDEN MYLK

INGREDIENTS

1/2 cup rolled oats (40.5g)
1/2 cup water (118.5g)
1/2 tablespoon turmeric (3.4g)
1/2 teaspoon black pepper (3.5g)
1 tablespoon coconut oil (13.6g)
1/4 teaspoon ground ginger (0.5g)
2 tablespoons honey (42g)

PREPARATION

1. Combine the rolled oats and water in a blender, and blend on high until completely smooth and creamy.
2. Add the turmeric, black pepper, coconut oil, ginger, and honey to the blender and blend on high for 1 minute, or until smooth. The consistency should be thin enough to drink through a straw. Add additional water to adjust the consistency if required.
3. Taste the mixture. If it is not sweet enough, add 1 teaspoon of honey or another sweetener, blend for 10-15 seconds, and taste.
4. When the mixture has reached the proper taste and consistency, pour into a large cup and enjoy.

NOTES:

NICK'S NUTRITIONAL NUGGETS

CURCUMIN & TURMERIC

Curcumin is the active ingredient in turmeric; curcumin is a very strong antioxidant with powerful anti-inflammatory effects.

Curcumin is fat-soluble and poorly absorbed into the bloodstream. Therefore, for maximal absorption and benefits, consume curcumin with black pepper and fatty meals.

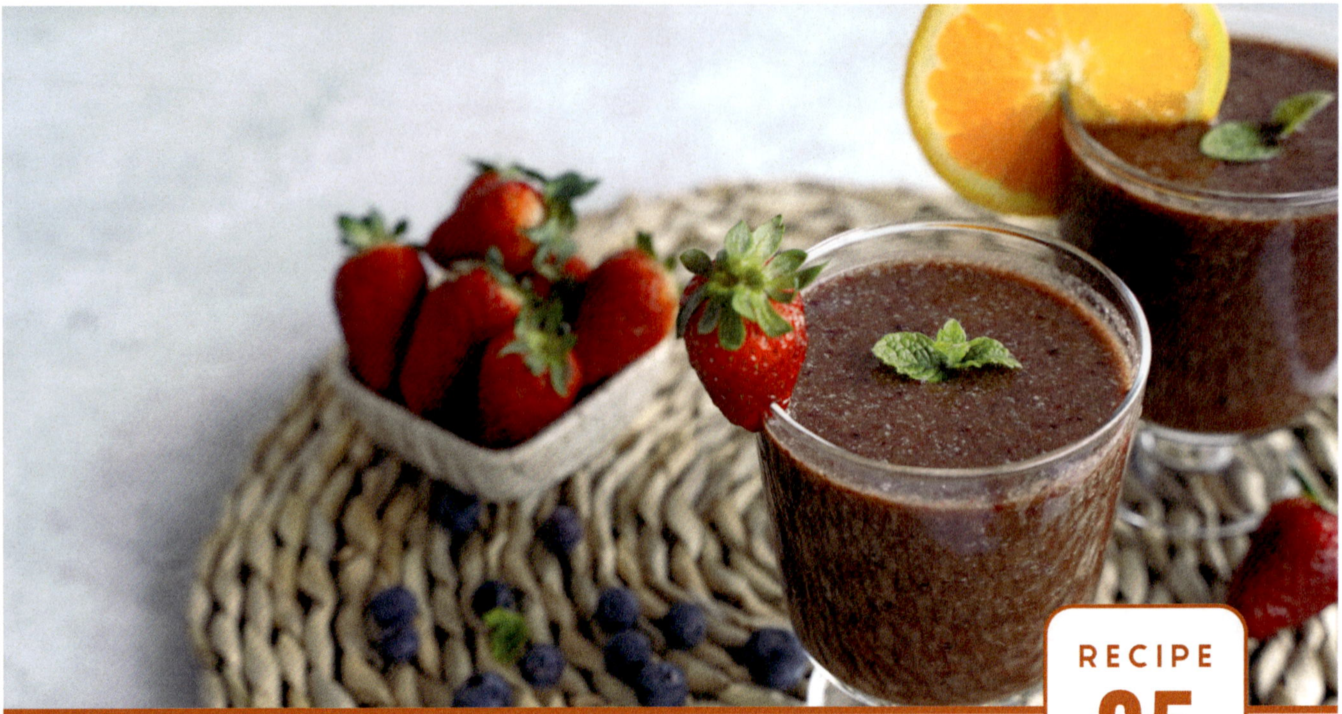

RECIPE 05

TROPICAL SLUSH

INGREDIENTS

1 cup crushed ice (236g)
1½ cups pulp-free orange juice (372g)
2 cups roughly chopped kale (134g)
2 cups chopped pineapple (330g)
1/2 cup chopped peaches (77g)
1 cup mixed berries (140g)
1½ tablespoons coconut oil (20.4g)
1 tablespoon honey (21g)

PREPARATION

1. Add all ingredients to a blender and blend on high for 1 minute, or until the mixture is a “slushy” consistency.
2. The consistency should be thin and smooth enough to drink through a straw, with some small chunks of ice throughout. Add additional ice or orange juice to adjust consistency.
3. Taste the mixture. If it is not sweet enough, add honey or another sweetener, blend for 10-15 seconds, and taste.
4. When the mixture has reached the proper taste and consistency, pour into a large cup and enjoy.

NOTES:

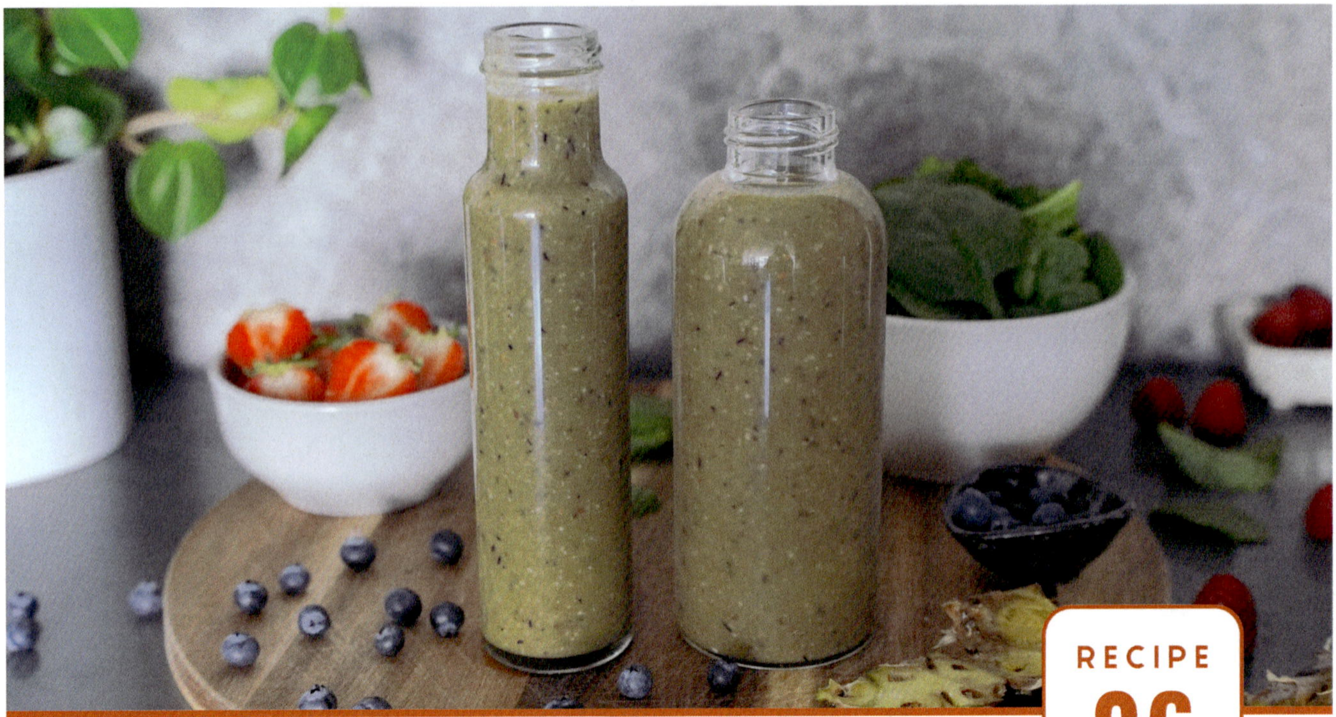

RECIPE 06

BERRY BLAST SLUSH

INGREDIENTS

2 cups spinach (60g)
2 cups chopped pineapple (330g)
1/2 cup blueberries (74g)
1/2 cup raspberries (61.5g)
1/2 cup chopped mango (82.5g)
1/2 cup strawberries (83g)
1½ tablespoons shredded dried sweetened coconut (21.3g)
1 tablespoon honey (21g)
1 cup crushed ice (236g)
4 oz. unsweetened vanilla almond milk - optional (113.4g)

PREPARATION

1. Add all ingredients to a blender and blend on high for 1 minute, or until the mixture is a "slushy" consistency.
2. The consistency should be thin and smooth enough to drink through a straw, with some small chunks of ice throughout. Add additional ice or almond milk to adjust the consistency if required.
3. Taste the mixture. If it is not sweet enough, add honey or another sweetener to taste, blend for 10-15 seconds, and taste.
4. When the mixture has reached the proper taste and consistency, pour into a large cup and enjoy.

NOTES:

nutrition facts beverages

Smoothie - Apple Pie

Nutrition Facts

1 serving per container
Serving size **1 cup (8oz) (0.0g)**

Amount Per Serving	
Calories	**1090**
	% Daily Value*
Total Fat 31g	**40%**
Saturated Fat 8g	**40%**
Trans Fat 0g	
Cholesterol 25mg	**8%**
Sodium 115mg	**5%**
Total Carbohydrate 169g	**61%**
Dietary Fiber 35g	**125%**
Total Sugars 79g	
Includes 0g Added Sugars	**0%**
Protein 26g	
Vitamin D 0.1mcg	0%
Calcium 370mg	30%
Iron 6.4mg	35%
Potassium 2060mg	45%

* The % Daily Value (DV) tells you how much a nutrient in a serving of food contributes to a daily diet. 2,000 calories a day is used for general nutrition advice.

Smoothie - Thick & Sweet

Nutrition Facts

1 serving per container
Serving size **1 cup (8oz) (0.0g)**

Amount Per Serving	
Calories	**500**
	% Daily Value*
Total Fat 21g	**27%**
Saturated Fat 5g	**25%**
Trans Fat 0g	
Polyunsaturated Fat 5g	
Monounsaturated Fat 10g	
Cholesterol 5mg	**2%**
Sodium 55mg	**2%**
Total Carbohydrate 62g	**23%**
Dietary Fiber 10g	**36%**
Total Sugars 25g	
Includes 18g Added Sugars	**36%**
Protein 26g	
Vitamin D 0mcg	0%
Calcium 180mg	15%
Iron 3.9mg	20%
Potassium 660mg	15%

* The % Daily Value (DV) tells you how much a nutrient in a serving of food contributes to a daily diet. 2,000 calories a day is used for general nutrition advice.

Smoothie - Mean Green

Nutrition Facts

1 serving per container
Serving size **1 cup (8oz) (0.0g)**

Amount Per Serving	
Calories	**950**
	% Daily Value*
Total Fat 24g	**31%**
Saturated Fat 6g	**30%**
Trans Fat 0g	
Cholesterol 0mg	**0%**
Sodium 100mg	**4%**
Total Carbohydrate 169g	**61%**
Dietary Fiber 29g	**104%**
Total Sugars 102g	
Includes 0g Added Sugars	**0%**
Protein 15g	
Vitamin D 0mcg	0%
Calcium 150mg	10%
Iron 4mg	20%
Potassium 1440mg	30%

* The % Daily Value (DV) tells you how much a nutrient in a serving of food contributes to a daily diet. 2,000 calories a day is used for general nutrition advice.

Smoothie - Golden Mylk

Nutrition Facts

1 serving per container
Serving size **1 cup (8oz) (0.0g)**

Amount Per Serving	
Calories	**420**
	% Daily Value*
Total Fat 16g	**21%**
Saturated Fat 12g	**60%**
Trans Fat 0g	
Polyunsaturated Fat 1g	
Monounsaturated Fat 1.5g	
Cholesterol 0mg	**0%**
Sodium 10mg	**0%**
Total Carbohydrate 67g	**24%**
Dietary Fiber 6g	**21%**
Total Sugars 35g	
Includes 34g Added Sugars	**68%**
Protein 6g	
Vitamin D 0mcg	0%
Calcium 50mg	4%
Iron 4.2mg	25%
Potassium 290mg	6%

* The % Daily Value (DV) tells you how much a nutrient in a serving of food contributes to a daily diet. 2,000 calories a day is used for general nutrition advice.

Tropical Slush

Nutrition Facts

1 serving per container
Serving size **8 oz (0.0g)**

Amount Per Serving	
Calories	**750**
	% Daily Value*
Total Fat 23g	**29%**
Saturated Fat 17g	**85%**
Trans Fat 0g	
Cholesterol 0mg	**0%**
Sodium 60mg	**3%**
Total Carbohydrate 135g	**49%**
Dietary Fiber 17g	**61%**
Total Sugars 100g	
Includes 17g Added Sugars	**34%**
Protein 12g	
Vitamin D 0mcg	0%
Calcium 310mg	25%
Iron 5mg	30%
Potassium 1920mg	40%

* The % Daily Value (DV) tells you how much a nutrient in a serving of food contributes to a daily diet. 2,000 calories a day is used for general nutrition advice.

Berry Blast Slush

Nutrition Facts

1 serving per container
Serving size **8 oz (0.0g)**

Amount Per Serving	
Calories	**510**
	% Daily Value*
Total Fat 11g	**14%**
Saturated Fat 7g	**35%**
Trans Fat 0g	
Cholesterol 0mg	**0%**
Sodium 200mg	**9%**
Total Carbohydrate 110g	**40%**
Dietary Fiber 16g	**57%**
Total Sugars 85g	
Includes 25g Added Sugars	**50%**
Protein 7g	
Vitamin D 1.2mcg	6%
Calcium 360mg	30%
Iron 4.5mg	25%
Potassium 1270mg	25%

* The % Daily Value (DV) tells you how much a nutrient in a serving of food contributes to a daily diet. 2,000 calories a day is used for general nutrition advice.

NICHOLAS KELLY:
A JOURNEY OF FLAVOR, RESILIENCE, AND NUTRITION

Nicholas Kelly embodies more than just the roles of dietitian, author, and advocate; he represents a saga of resilience. Diagnosed with cystic fibrosis at three months old, he has never let this condition define him. Instead, it spurred a lifelong dedication to impactful living and culinary exploration.

Nicholas's culinary odyssey started in his family's kitchen, blossoming into an intense passion for crafting meals that delight and nourish. Untrained yet innately skilled, his inventive approach focuses on high-calorie dishes designed to enrich both body and soul.

The genesis of his cookbook was a blend of empathy and necessity, driven by a conversation highlighting the scarcity of enjoyable, nutritious high-calorie meals. This seven-year endeavor was fraught with challenges but underscored by Nicholas's unwavering commitment to his vision and health.

What distinguishes Nicholas's cookbook is its comprehensive nutritional insights, coupled with delicious recipes. It's a testament to his belief in the possibility of gourmet, high-calorie eating that's both satisfying and healthful.

Nicholas's narrative is not just about culinary success but a personal testament to perseverance and the power of following one's passions. His hope for readers is to find joy and nourishment in his recipes, fostering a new appreciation for high-calorie cuisine.

For more about Nicholas's journey, advocacy, and culinary philosophy, visit www.NicholasKellyRD.com.

Made in United States
Orlando, FL
04 November 2026

90200577R00071